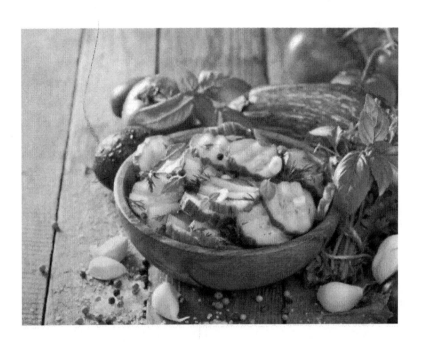

Renal Diet Coockbook

By Antony J. Willfour and Sandy J Zogheib

*T*his document is geared towards providing exact and reliable information in regards to the topic and issue covered. The publication is sold with the idea that the publisher is not required to render accounting, officially permitted, or otherwise, qualified services. If advice is necessary, legal or professional, a practiced individual in the profession should be ordered.

- From a Declaration of Principles which was accepted and approved equally by a Committee of the American Bar Association and a Committee of Publishers and Associations.

the information provided herein is stated to be truthful and consistent, in that any liability, in terms of inattention or otherwise, by any usage or abuse of any policies, processes, or directions contained within is the solitary and utter responsibility of the recipient reader. Under no circumstances will any legal responsibility or blame be held against the publisher for any reparation, damages, or monetary loss due to the information herein, either directly or indirectly.

Respective authors own all copyrights not held by the publisher.

The information herein is offered for informational purposes solely, and is universal as so. The presentation of the information is without contract or any type of guarantee assurance.

The trademarks that are used are without any consent and the publication of the trademark is without permission or backing by the trademark owner. All trademarks and brands within this book are for clarifying purposes only and are the owned by the owners themselves, not affiliated with this document.

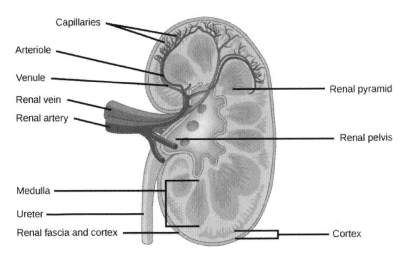

Capillaries

Arteriole

Venule

Renal vein

Renal artery

Renal pyramid

Renal pelvis

Medulla

Ureter

Renal fascia and cortex

Cortex

Reanal Structure

Table of Contents

INTRODUCTION

A Renal diet is an eating plan worked out to help people suffering from renal diseases to boost the effectiveness of treatment by minimizing the levels of waste products in their blood.

The renal diet is designed to cause as little extra work or stress on the damaged kidneys as possible, while still providing sufficient good nutrients and energy that the body needs.

A renal diet follows several basic guidelines. The first guideline is that it must be a balanced, healthy and sustainable diet, rich in fibers, vitamins, natural grains, carbohydrates, omega 3 fats, and fluids. Proteins should be adequate, but not excessive.

The salts that are likely to accumulate in the bloodstream, are kept to a minimum. Blood electrolyte levels are monitored regularly and the diet adjusted accordingly. It is very important to follow specific advice from your doctor and dietitian.

+ Daily protein intake is important to rebuild tissues but should be kept to a minimum. Superfluous proteins need to be broken down by the body into carbohydrates and nitrates. Nitrates are not used by the body and have to be excreted through the kidneys.

+ Carbohydrates are an important source of energy and should be taken in adequate quantities. Whole grains and unrefined forms of carbohydrates are the best. Avoid highly refined carbohydrates.

+ Table salt should be restricted to cooking only. Excess salt causes fluid retention and stresses the kidneys. Salty foods such as processed meats; sausages, many tinned foods, and snacks should be avoided.

17

✦ Phosphorus is essential for the body to function properly, but dialysis cannot remove it, so levels need to be monitored carefully and intake should be limited though not eliminated.

✦ Foods such as dairy products, legumes and darker colored drinks like colas, have high phosphorus contents. Foods high in the potassium content, such as dark leafy green vegetables, bananas, apricots, and citrus fruits, might also need to be restricted if blood levels rise.

✦ Omega 3 fats are an important part of any healthy diet. Fatty fish is an excellent source. Omega fats are essential for healthy body functioning. Avoid trans-fats or hydrolyzed fats.

✦ Fluids should be adequate but might need to be restricted in cases of fluid retention.

A healthy renal diet can help retain kidney function for longer. The main differences between any healthy diet and a renal diet, are the restrictions placed on protein and table salt intake.

Restrictions on phosphorus, potassium, and fluids may become necessary as symptoms and signs of accumulation become evident.

Every information in this renal diet cookbook, are intended to help keep kidney sufferers healthy and functional by eating to support and augment their treatment. Also are quick and easy to prepare renal recipes. It is very important to get specific advice from your doctor and dietitian at all times.

LOW PROTEIN RENAL DIET - HOW TO EFFECTIVELY USE IT TO REVERSE KIDNEY DISEASE PROGRESSION

The low protein renal diet controls the intake of fluid, protein, sodium, potassium, and phosphorus. One question that is often asked about this kidney diet is whether the protein is allowed or not. Well, the answer is that it depends upon the status of your kidneys.

The number of nutrients in the diet is based on your blood levels of sodium, potassium, phosphorus, calcium, albumin, and urea. These levels are measured before and immediately after a dialysis treatment.

Fluid restriction is based on the amount of urine output and weight gain between dialysis treatments. That is, whatever goes out of your body in liquid form has to be replaced with water.

Monitoring and taking note of your daily weight would be a good practice to indicate fluid retention which suggests kidney deterioration.

Preservation of renal function can delay the need for dialysis therapy. It can be accomplished by controlling the disease process, by controlling blood pressure and by reducing dietary protein intake and catabolism.

A kidney patient's low protein renal diet depends on specific adjustments of dietary elements through the results of the client's blood chemistry studies. Although there is some debate over whether and how to restrict proteins, keeping the daily intake of protein of high biologic value below 50 g may slow the progression of renal failure.

The amount of protein you can eat is based on how well your kidneys are functioning and the amount of protein needed to maintain good health. When protein is used by the body, waste products are formed and enter the blood. One of these wastes is called urea. Normal healthy kidneys are good at getting rid of urea. Failing kidneys are not good at this, but kidney patients should still eat protein.

As the renal disease progresses, the client's ability and willingness to take in adequate nutrition diminish and the challenge becomes not only to maintain appropriate intake of non-protein calories but also to satisfy protein needs. In these instances, elemental diets, enteral feedings or total parenteral nutrition may be used instead of or in addition to regular food intake. This is why kidney dialysis diet is so important in order for patients to follow a proper balance of electrolytes, minerals, and fluid in patients who are on dialysis.

Low protein renal diet should be done with the approval of your health care provider. In fact, your health care provider would be so proud of you for taking a proactive approach to managing your kidney disease. Remember, ignorance is never an excuse for bad health habits.

RENAL DIET GUIDELINES

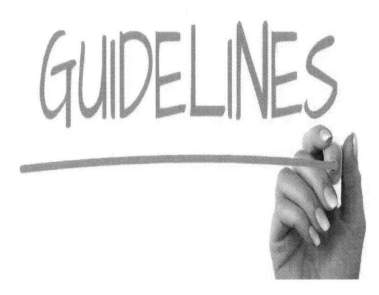

here is no one specific "renal diet", only guidelines to help you control the levels of salts in your bloodstream through what you eat. The diet required for renal deficiency varies with each case, the severity of the malfunction, whether the swelling is present, whether you are overweight, what your blood electrolyte readings are, and whether you are a candidate for dialysis or not.

With renal failure, the salts in the bloodstream are completely thrown off balance. The aim of renal diet guidelines is to help control the build-up of waste products and fluid in your blood by placing less pressure on your kidneys.

Renal diet guidelines are built around blood test results and a normal healthy balanced diet. The idea is to limit the intake of salts that are too high. Fluids may also be restricted if your kidneys are unable to excrete sufficient water. Protein intake is limited so wastes like urea are kept at a minimum.

The salts that commonly need to be restricted are:

Sodium. Sodium can cause high blood pressure and fluid retention.

Most renal diets use minimal salt in cooking, and stipulate, "No added salts". "Lo-salt" combinations are not suitable for salt replacement as they have high potassium levels, and should not be used. Processed foods, sausages, sauces, ketchup's and many canned foods should be avoided.

Phosphorus cannot be removed by dialysis, so it might become a problem. Levels are monitored, and kept under control by diet and sometimes medication. High phosphorus foods include dairy products, beans, peas, beer and cola drinks.

Potassium should only be restricted if the blood levels are high.

Many healthy vegetables and fruits contain potassium. High potassium foods include apricots, orange juice, bananas, avocados, beets, spinach and many more.

Proteins are a necessary part of a healthy diet, but should only be eaten in small amounts. Proteins that should be restricted, include all meats, fish, eggs and dairy products.

Fluids might be restricted if water retention is present in the form of generalized swelling or fluid in the lungs. Fluids are often strictly controlled for patients' on hemodialysis. Fluids include all beverages, soups, water, and juices.

Carbohydrates are energy foods and should not be restricted unless you are diabetic or overweight. Lastly, it might be advisable to take vitamin and antioxidant supplements to boost your immune system.

Benefits of A Healthy Renal Diet To Kidney Disease Patient
This article discusses the benefits of a renal diet to a patient whose kidneys are malfunctioning due to kidney disease.

It is the role of your kidneys to filter out things you don't need and to maintain a balance of the good things your body needs. If your kidneys can't play this role efficiently what can you do to get toxic substances from your body? A Doctor recommended renal diet could help you filter out toxic substances you don't need in your body.

A healthy renal diet can indeed help you to manage this problem.

The aim of the Doctor is to help you filter toxic substances long before they get in your body. Toxic substances get into your body through the food you eat. If you can avoid eating foods that contain toxic substances you will be able to lessen the burden on your kidneys to flash out unwanted things from your bloodstream.

The benefit of following a healthy diet is feeling good and having more energy   A healthy renal diet means less taxation of your kidneys:

Apart from eliminating urine and other toxic substances such as ammonia, your kidneys help the body to create red blood cells and to keep blood pressure steady. A Doctor recommended diet ensures your kidneys have a lesser workload to handle. This happens through the control of toxic substances intake. Some of the leading substances that add toxins in your bloodstream and cause problems for your kidneys are; sodium, potassium, some proteins, and phosphorous. A Doctor monitored dietary regime will ensure that these substances are eliminated completely from your diet or they are taken in moderation.

A renal diet helps you to prevent the progression of renal failure.

You want to make sure that your kidney problem does not develop into kidney failure. A healthy diet as recommended by your doctor plays a major role in the management of your kidney disease such that it doesn't grow out of control.

A Renal Diet Helps in the Control of Phosphorous and Potassium Levels in your Body:

A healthy diet helps you to limit protein to the right amount and to maintain bone strength by making sure there isn't too much phosphorous in your bloodstream. It also ensures that there is no excess potassium in your system because it can adversely affect your heartbeat.

A renal diet ensures that the level of sodium in your body is under strict control in order to avoid water retention. If fluids are retained in your body as a result of excessive sodium intake, you shall suffer a lot of pain due to swellings around leg joints.

KIDNEY DIET

If you suffer from kidney disease, what can you eat when following the kidney diet plan? A lowphosphoric diet is recommended because when your kidneys are experiencing problems, then you begin to have phosphorus levels that are too high. To avoid further health issues, you must limit your phosphorus intake. Most of the kidney diet foods are simply a matter of substituting one food for another.

Here are some examples:

✦ Substitute dairy products for non-dairy products. Skip the milk and drink unfortified rice milk.

✦ Cream cheese or cottage cheese instead of hard cheeses.

✦ Refined grains instead of whole grains.

The top fifteen foods that will benefit a person who suffers from kidney disease, include these starchy vegetables: potatoes, rutabagas, and winter squash rather than corn, parsnips, pumpkin, or sweet potatoes. Other vegetables include red peppers, cabbage, cauliflower, garlic, and onions. Some fruits are apples, cranberries, blueberries, raspberries, strawberries, cherries, and red grapes. Also, egg whites, fish, and olive oil are listed in the top fifteen too.

Basically, in order to consume kidney diet foods, you need to know which foods contain more or less phosphorus. Manufacturers have a way of hiding phosphorus in additives and you must learn which to look for and take notice of these when you are grocery shopping.

Some examples of these are calcium phosphate, disodium phosphate, phosphoric acid, and other types containing the word polyphosphates. These manufacturers are not required to consider your health and list the amount of phosphorus in each product so you must learn to recognize them for yourself.

An important measure to take for yourself is to consult a dietitian who understands your specific needs. He or she will be able to help you come up with a meal plan geared toward kidney diet foods. Your goal is to maintain your health the best you can despite having kidney disease. The key is to control the amount of phosphorus that your body takes in.

Diet Tips to Effectively Combat Renal Failure

Before dealing about the changes that are necessary to combat renal failure, it will be helpful to know that this illness is not the only health complaint most of the times. There are a few other complications such as diabetes or heart ailment that lay hidden in many patients for a long time.

In such a case, a diet known as the ketogenic meal schedule is prescribed, which includes items that are low in carbohydrate content and high in terms of specially prepared fat. In addition, such a specialized type of food menu ensures that your body gets the right amount of essential nutrients to make sure that the road to recovery is safe and steady.

In fact, these patients can hope to postpone dialysis for some time if their body accepts the changes and responds positively.

This should encourage you to continue with home-made remedies to deal with and heal renal malfunctioning or failure in an utmost effective manner.

A few other popular items that are prescribed for patients diagnosed with renal failure are:

A. Fruits like pineapple and berries like cranberry, raspberry, blueberry, and strawberry

B. Tea varieties such as Java tea and green tea

C. Herbal extracts from

- Rehmannia

- Cough grass

- Uva ursi

A. Items low in animal fat and protein

B. Grape seeds and extracts

What are the special features of a kidney diet?

True to its growing popularity, this type of diet schedule is being recommended by medical practitioners and dieticians across the world. A few examples of an average day of this plan will be something like:

a. Egg whites included and the yellow parts excluded

b. Lean meat included and red meat excluded

c. Fish included but only certain varieties that are low in fat and that too in a very small quantity only

d. Inclusion of carbohydrate items only up to 8 grams per day

e. Fresh fruits like citrus fruits as they contain less level of sugar and also minimum fleshy content

f. Even the cereals, grains and condiments included in your diet should be whole since they have low-fat content

g. Vegetables like asparagus, onion, cabbage, parsley, and sprouted kidney beans

h. Items made in olive or flaxseed oil

Generally, in this type of diet, there is a recommended diet formula on a per-day basis, which includes the various elements like calcium, phosphorus, potassium, protein, fluids, sodium, etc.

Interestingly, the nature of the diet recommendations varies according to the severity and the present condition of the failure of the renal system.

KIDNEY DIET SECRETS - NEW WAYS TO OVERCOME YOUR KIDNEY PROBLEMS

People who suffer from kidney disease can rejoice-they won't have to worry about restricting food intake or live with restricting questionable foods anymore. This diet helps ensure the survivability of their kidneys, in addition to keeping the rest of their body smoothly running. The diet we're talking about is no secret - it's called the renal or kidney diet.

The term renal refers to anything involving the kidneys, hence the alternative name renal diet. These diets typically get prescribed to kidney patients, according to how much their condition has progressed.

If you're suffering from kidney failure, it's best to consult with your doctor or dietitian about what kind of kidney diet you'll need to consume on a daily basis. Kidney diets are formulated to control the essential minerals and nutrients of the body.

So, what are the secrets to managing your kidney diet? To start, when your kidney disease progresses into later stages, you will have to stop consuming certain amounts of:

- Fluids.
- Phosphorus. ▪ Potassium.

In addition, some not so secretive things you need to know, in regards to your diet include:

- Managing alkaline levels, which help nourish your weakened kidneys.
- Avoiding fluids that either "contaminate" the kidneys, deprive the body of fluids and nutrients, or impair the entire body, especially if you've consumed a lot.

Remaining dedicated to your diet.

You'll also need to stop consuming certain foods like red meats, various dairy products, alcohol, many gluten-based products, highly processed foods, and sugar. These foods can negatively affect your kidneys if you're suffering from kidney failure, causing other problems for your kidneys and surrounding organs.

You can, however, add the following foods to your kidney diet:

+ Fruits- peaches, pears, apples, pineapples, blueberries, grapes.
+ Vegetables-cabbage, mushrooms, radishes, iceberg lettuce, cauliflower.
+ Proteins-chicken, tofu and some types of fish.
+ Other foods-white rice, olives, hummus, macadamia nuts, flaxseed oil.

Once you've sorted out your dietary essentials, you'll have started monitoring your intakes of nutrients and minerals, like your sodium and proteins. A doctor or dietitian can help you figure out how much of each nutrient and minerals you need to consume within your diet.

One of the best kidney diet secrets involves getting your blood tested, which lets you find out how much nutrients and minerals you actually need. If you get your blood tested, you and a doctor will be able to determine the number of nutrients and minerals you need in your daily diet. Remember-staying on track when undertaking a kidney diet ensures the health of your kidneys.

KIDNEY DISEASE - DIET FOR KIDNEY FAILURE

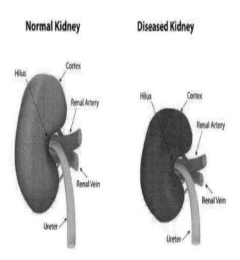

Diet kidney is a term that is used to describe the special diet which must be adhered to by people with a failed or diseased kidney. One of the most recurring complaints is that this diet type has too many constraints and tends to be very strict and relentless.

What Is Kidney Failure

The kidney is a major player in the regulation of human bodily functions. Apart from aiding the body in getting rid of its wastes, it also helps in filtering the blood, stimulating the production of red blood cells and creates a balance in the level of electrolytes in the body. Kidney failure thereby occurs with the inability of the kidneys to perform the aforementioned functions.

Kidney failure is an almost endemic condition that can be a common conduit for different renal and urinary tract diseases. If it gets worse, wastes can build up to high and dangerous levels in your blood, thereby causing complications which can include; nerve damage, poor nutritional health, high blood pressure, and anemia.

Importance of Good Nutrition For Diet Kidney

A good and balanced diet is essential for people with damaged or deteriorating kidney functions. Eating healthy is important to everyone but is even more so to people with kidney failure. Only good nutrition can give you the energy you need to do your daily tasks, maintain a healthy weight, help build muscles and prevent infections. Consultations with your physician can help in understanding what foods may or may not be appropriate, if extra nutrients need to be taken, and most probably, a referral to a dietician who can work out a diet plan for you.

The Basics of A Good Diet For Kidney Disease

The basics of a healthy nutritional eating plan are to devise a plan which gives the recipient the right amount of Calories, Protein, Minerals, and Vitamins.

PROTEIN: Getting the right amount of protein is paramount to your overall health and wellbeing. Some of the most important sources of protein are Red Meat(veal, lamb, beef), Poultry, Eggs, Fish and other seafood, Pork, Grains, and Vegetables.

CALORIES: Calories are like the fuel our body needs to produce energy with which we carry out our everyday activities. They help in maintaining healthy body weight and allows the body to use up protein to repair the muscles and tissues in the body. The amount of calories our body needs differs from one individual to the other. If you are not getting the right amount of calories in your diet, you may need to eat extra high sugary foods like jam, syrup, honey, hard candy, etc.

MINERALS and VITAMINS: As a result of kidney disease and dialysis, the number of minerals and vitamins your body needs changes.

Because you are on a special diet, the limit on your food choices can deprive you of many of the important minerals and vitamins you would otherwise get from various food sources. Therefore, you may need to take special vitamins or minerals as recommended by your physician ONLY.

Controlling Other Important Nutrients

If you suffer from kidney disease, you may need to balance fluids and other essential minerals and electrolytes which can have a big impact on your day to day living. These include:

PHOSPHORUS: Found in dairy products, nuts, bran, and beverages.

Too much phosphorus in the body can result in weak bones, a build-up of calcium in the heart, blood vessels, joints, and muscles. This can ultimately lead to heart conditions, skin ulcers, and poor blood circulation.

POTASSIUM: The amount of potassium you need depends on many factors which can include any medication that can alter the levels of potassium in the body. Too much or too little can be dangerous because some people on dialysis may need more potassium while others may be less. Good sources include leafy green vegetables, banana, avocado, milk, dried beans, and peas, etc. **CALCIUM:** Is the key mineral for building strong bones. Moreover, there is a high phosphorus content in foods that are good sources of calcium. To counter this setback, you may need to take phosphate binders and a special form of vitamin D which can be recommended by your physician.

SODIUM: This affects blood pressure and water balance in your body. Sodium is found in table salt, seasoning, canned foods, and processed meats. Lack of sodium can lead to swelling of the ankle, fingers, and eyes.

The kidney has a remarkable ability to recover from certain conditions if diagnosed early and treated using dialysis, diet, and or transplantation.

Potassium Diet - A Low Potassium Diet for Kidney Disease If you are someone that suffers from weakened or diseased kidneys, then you need to be very careful about the foods you eat. A good kidney Diet plan will help you to keep an eye on minerals like potassium and calcium that can easily start to build up in the body due to the kidneys being unable to rid the body of them in time. Getting too much potassium can lead to a problem called hyperkalemia, which involves having too high of a concentration of potassium in the blood. If you suffer from kidney problems, you will need to watch how much potassium you get each day to avoid this.

Normally, it is recommended people get around 4700 mg potassium each day. For those that are suffering from a chronic kidney disease that amount should be no more than 2700 mg. To stay within these boundaries, a good kidney Diet plan should consist of things like three servings of vegetables and three servings of fruits that are low in potassium each day, such as lettuce, cucumbers, and apples. A dairy is a good option because it is low in potassium and the calcium it has is easy for the body to absorb. Try to get one or two servings of dairy each day. This can include things like cheddar cheese and a small amount of margarine.

A good kidney Diet plan will usually contain between three and seven servings of meats that are low in potassium each day. Turkey breast is always a healthy choice, and you can have a hardboiled egg as well. When it comes to grains, between four and seven servings will be fine. Some good foods that fall into the grain category that are also low in potassium include white bread, English muffins, and unsweetened corn cereal.

A good low potassium diet can still involve you enjoying all or most of your favorite vegetables. The only recommendation is that you LEACH the vegetables before consumption. The process of leaching will help pull potassium out of some high-potassium vegetables. However, you should bear in mind that leaching will not pull out all of the potassium from your vegetables.

Once you get accustomed to a good Kidney Diet plan that is low in potassium you will see that it's not terribly challenging to follow. As long as you avoid fruits like bananas and kiwis that are very high in potassium and make sure to drink enough fluids, you should be in good shape.

KIDNEY DIET - 5 TIPS FOR A HEALTHY KIDNEY DIET

A kidney diet helps kidneys maintain optimal performance.

Maintaining a good renal diet extends the usefulness and well-being of the kidneys and the individual concerned. Kidney diets become more important when kidneys are diseased or malfunctioning.

Kidneys are small organs that act as filters in our body. Their main function is to purify and cleanse our blood. This is accomplished by the removal of excess water, toxins and other harmful waste products. Together they constitute what

45

is known as urine which is then passed to the bladder. In time, urine is removed through urination.

If kidneys do not function well, severe body disorders and possibly death could be the result. Symptoms such as blood poisoning, water retention, reduced blood cell production (anemia), lethargy and fatigue are some of the main discomforts of kidney failure. Therefore one should always try to stick to a healthy kidney diet so as to lead a healthy life and prevent kidney disease. Here are 5 tips for a healthy kidney diet:

1. Cut down on fatty foods to reduce cholesterol. In addition to minimizing kidney disease, you also reduce the possibility of heart attacks and strokes.

2. Reduce obesity by watching your calories. Live a healthy lifestyle by doing more physical exercise, less over-eating, and other healthy activities. Additionally, you also avoid other distasteful and life-threatening sicknesses.

3. Table salt intake should be avoided completely or greatly reduced. Table salt is known to increase blood pressure and put pressure on the kidneys to work harder.

4. Drink more water as this helps the kidneys to perform better.

5. Finally, put away dark colas, spirits, and alcohol or at least reduce the amount you consume.

And how do you benefit by doing all these?

None of the above requires a higher budget so a healthy renal diet is very possible. All supermarkets stock these food items mentioned above, close to where you live. Exercising can be obtained using free or paid methods. Going for walks is free so is running in the street. Using a gym or buying a treadmill requires money. The choice is yours. Willpower is needed and the urge to start and continue exercising. Nothing drastic, just 30 minutes a day is what most doctors recommend. There is really no excuse not to follow healthy kidney diets.

Kidney Diet - Help Kidneys By Controlling Protein, Fluids, Phosphorous, Potassium and Sodium Intake

The kidney diet often referred to as the renal diet is designed for people with kidney disease. Over 31 million people here in the US have kidney disease and the numbers are increasing. Medical professionals such as doctors and hospitals working with kidney disease patients developed this special eating plan with the medical science community and are based on scientific research.

There is no single kidney diet as each plan is specific to each person. This requires careful research and monitoring in order to design the correct plan for each patient's needs. The patient needs to work with a renal dietitian to get the right eating plan to fit their dietary requirements. This is based on information such as age, activity, if they are on dialysis and the degree of kidney failure. There are strict guidelines to control the amount of protein, fluids, phosphorous, potassium and sodium that are consumed, and this helps the kidneys.

Protein is an element that should be monitored. Protein is needed to repair, maintain and build muscles, glands, and organs. When protein is used by the body it creates urea. Urea is a waste product that is filtered from the body in urine by the kidneys.

When the kidneys are not working properly, urea can build up and could cause other serious illness. Controlling the amount and type of protein consumed is necessary to extend the health of the kidneys.

Fluids both the type and the amount can be a major concern depending upon how much kidney function there is.

Phosphorus and potassium are two other minerals that are found in high amounts in many different foods, such as fruits, vegetables, nuts, colas, and dairy foods. These minerals are also necessary for bodily functions. The kidneys task is to regulate the amount of these minerals that are in the body. Having an overabundance of phosphorus can cause bone loss and too much potassium can adversely affect the heart. Most salt substitutes are made of potassium chloride and are not allowed on most kidney diets. Many low sodium products are now being made with potassium chloride.

You must pay attention to this to help avoid too much potassium in your diet.

Sodium is important to many bodily functions and can be found in abundance in our foods, especially processed food, fast food, and restaurant food. One important function that sodium controls the amount of fluid in the body. With a high level of sodium in the body, thirst is increased and fluids buildup. The kidneys help to keep the amount of sodium in the body at the correct levels. Too much sodium intake can put unneeded pressure on the kidneys. Too much sodium has been proven and linked to increased blood pressure. Controlling blood pressure is of major importance to help the kidneys and prevent further damage from kidney disease.

Simply stop adding extra salt to your food at the table or while cooking will help to significantly reduce sodium intake. Many people add salt to their food at the table out of habit, and just by removing the salt shakers can help eliminate that habit. Don't cook with salt. Use herbs and spices instead. It is also important to stay away from salty foods like potato chips, salted popcorn, processed cheese, and bacon, ham or any other cured meats. Often canned, frozen, and processed foods are loaded with sodium. It is important to check the ingredients of these foods for their sodium content. Canned soups are one of those foods that can have an enormous amount of sodium. There are now many brands with lower sodium versions. Be aware these may still be fairly high in sodium especially for kidney patients and may be made with potassium chloride instead of salt.

With so many people relying on salt to add flavor to food, it is smart to discover a replacement for it. Many choose natural salt substitutes like fresh lemon juice or vinegar. They may find a specific herb or spice like black pepper, as a flavor they like and use it to add flavor instead of salt. There are a number of salt-free seasonings without potassium chloride available that will safely create more flavorful low sodium meals while following the kidney diet.

4 WEEKS KIDNEY DIALYSIS DIET - DAILY TIPS TO BOOST YOUR KIDNEY FUNCTION AT

WEEK 1

DAY 1

Sweet Asian Beef Stir-Fry

This Asian-inspired beef stir-fry recipe is loaded with crisp-tender vegetables and served over spaghetti with a sweet orange-teriyaki sauce. If you don't have spaghetti noodles in your pantry, substitute soba noodles, rice or quinoa

Ingredients

4 servings

3 tablespoons low-sugar orange marmalade2 tablespoons light teriyaki sauce2 tablespoons water1 tablespoon grated fresh ginger¼ to ½ teaspoon crushed red pepper3 ounces dried multigrain spaghetti or soba (buckwheat) noodlesNonstick cooking spray2 cups small broccoli florets½ of a small red onion, cut into thin wedges1 cup packaged julienned carrots, or 2 carrots, cut into thin bite-size strips2 teaspoons canola oil12 ounces boneless beef top sirloin steak,

cut into thin bite-size strips (see Tip)3 cups shredded napa cabbage

Preparation

In a small bowl, combine marmalade, teriyaki sauce, the water, ginger and crushed red pepper; set aside. Cook spaghetti according to package directions. Meanwhile, coat a large nonstick skillet or wok with cooking spray. Preheat over medium-high heat. Add broccoli and red onion to hot skillet. Cover and cook for 3 minutes, stirring occasionally. Add carrots; cover and cook for 3 to 4 minutes more or until vegetables are crisp-tender, stirring occasionally. Remove vegetables from skillet. Add oil to the same skillet. Add beef strips. Cook and stir over medium-high heat for 3 to 5 minutes or until slightly pink in center. Return vegetables to skillet along with sauce and cabbage. Cook and stir for 1 to 2 minutes or until heated through and cabbage is just wilted. Serve immediately over the hot cooked spaghetti.

Tip: For easier slicing, partially freeze the steak before cutting it.

DAY 2

Pork Skewers **with** Fruit Glaze

Here's a quick and easy entree for six—chunks of succulent pork loin and red and green bell peppers are threaded onto skewers and grilled with a sweet fruit glaze. Choose your favorite fruit preserve for the glaze, like apricot, red raspberry, or strawberry.

Ingredients

6 servings

1 egg, slightly beaten⅓ cup finely chopped water chestnuts¼ cup fine dry breadcrumbs2 teaspoons grated fresh ginger1 clove garlic, minced¼ teaspoon salt¼ teaspoon ground pepper1 pound lean ground pork loin1 large red, yellow, or green bell pepper, cut into 1-inch pieces⅔ cup desired flavor low-sugar fruit preserves¼ cup pineapple juice1 tablespoon lemon juice¼ teaspoon ground cardamom

Preparation

Prep

30 m

Ready In

40 m

Combine egg, water chestnuts, breadcrumbs, ginger, garlic, salt, and ground pepper in a large bowl. Add ground pork; mix well. Shape the pork mixture into 30 meatballs. Alternately thread the meatballs and bell pepper pieces on six long metal skewers, leaving ¼ inch between pieces; set aside. Prepare glaze: place fruit preserves in a small saucepan; snip any large pieces. Stir in pineapple juice, lemon juice, and cardamom. Bring to boiling; reduce heat. Simmer, uncovered, for 15 minutes. Set aside to cool for 10 minutes while the pork cooks (the glaze will thicken as it cools). For a charcoal grill, arrange medium-hot coals around a drip pan. Test for medium heat above the pan. Place the skewers on well greased grill rack over the pan. Cover; grill for 10 to 12 minutes or until the meatballs are no longer pink and the juices run clear. Brush with some of the fruit glaze. Immediately remove the skewers from the grill. (For a gas grill, preheat grill. Reduce heat to medium. Adjust for indirect cooking. Grill as above.) Serve the skewers with the remaining glaze.

DAY 3

Red Cabbage-Apple Cauliflower Gnocchi

Tender cabbage and a vibrant applesauce-mustard pan sauce are the perfect pairing for pillowy low-carb cauliflower gnocchi. Add diced chicken-apple sausage for extra protein.

Ingredients

4 servings

3 cups shredded red cabbage2 tablespoons water, divided1 tablespoon olive oil1 (12 ounce) bag frozen cauliflower gnocchi½ cup unsweetened applesauce1 tablespoon Dijon mustardFreshly ground pepper to taste

Preparation

Place cabbage in a large microwave-safe bowl or baking dish. Add 1 tablespoon water. Cover tightly and microwave on High until softened, about 5 minutes. Heat oil in a large skillet over medium-high heat. Add gnocchi and cook, stirring frequently, until browned, about 5 minutes. Add cabbage and the remaining 1 tablespoon water; cover and cook, stirring occasionally, until the water evaporates. Stir in applesauce and mustard and heat through. Season with pepper.

DAY 4

Chicken-Spaghetti Squash Bake

In this version of a chicken-and-broccoli casserole, spaghetti squash takes on a creamy texture when baked with cream of mushroom soup.

Ingredients

8 servings

1 medium spaghetti squash (about 3 lbs.)4 cups broccoli florets1 tablespoon canola oil1 (10 ounce) package sliced mushrooms1 medium onion, finely chopped2 cloves garlic, minced½ teaspoon dried thyme½ teaspoon ground pepper2 (10 ounce) cans reduced-sodium condensed cream of mushroom soup, such as Campbell's 25% Less Sodium1½ pounds boneless, skinless chicken breasts, cut into bite-size pieces½ cup shredded extra-sharp Cheddar cheese

Preparation

Prep

55 m

Ready In

1 h 40 m

Preheat oven to 375°F. Coat two 8-inch-square baking dishes with cooking spray. Halve squash lengthwise and scoop out the seeds. Place cut-side down in a microwave-safe dish; add 2 Tbsp. water. Microwave, uncovered, on High until the flesh can be scraped with a fork but is still tender-crisp, 10 to 12 minutes. Scrape the strands onto a plate; set aside. Place broccoli in the same microwave-safe dish; add 1 Tbsp. water and cover. Microwave on High, stirring occasionally, until just barely tender-crisp, 2 to 3 minutes. Drain and set aside to cool. Meanwhile, heat oil in a large nonstick skillet over medium-high heat. Add mushrooms and cook, stirring, until they've released their juices, about 8 minutes. Add onion and continue cooking until the onion is tender and the mushrooms are lightly browned, about 8 minutes. Stir in garlic, thyme, and pepper; cook, stirring, for 30 seconds, Stir in soup (do not dilute with water) and heat through. Stir in chicken and the reserved squash and broccoli; gently toss to combine well. Divide the mixture between the prepared baking dishes and sprinkle each with ¼ cup Cheddar. Cover with foil. Label and freeze one casserole for up to 1 month. Bake the remaining casserole until bubbling, about 25 minutes. Uncover and continue baking until lightly browned along the edges, 10 to 15 minutes more. Let stand for 10 minutes before serving.

To make ahead: This double-batch recipe makes one casserole for tonight and one to freeze for up to 1 month (see Step 6). To cook from frozen: Thaw overnight in the refrigerator. Spoon off any liquid that has accumulated in the pan, if desired. Bake as directed in Step 7.

Equipment: Two 8-inch-square baking dishes or foil pans

DAY 5

Loaded Black Bean Nacho Soup

Jazz up a can of black bean soup with your favorite nacho toppings, such as cheese, avocado and fresh tomatoes. A bit of smoked paprika adds a bold flavor kick, but you can swap in any warm spices you prefer, such as cumin or chili powder.

Look for a soup that contains no more than 450 mg sodium per serving.

Ingredients

2 servings

1 (18 ounce) carton low-sodium black bean soup¼ teaspoon smoked paprika½ teaspoon lime juice½ cup halved grape tomatoes½ cup shredded cabbage or slaw mix2 tablespoons crumbled cotija cheese or other Mexican-style shredded cheese½ medium avocado, diced2 ounces baked tortilla chips

Preparation

Pour soup into a small saucepan and stir in paprika. Heat according to package directions. Stir in lime juice. Divide the soup between 2 bowls and top with tomatoes, cabbage (or slaw), cheese and avocado. Serve with tortilla chips.

DAY 6

Pesto Shrimp Pasta

Using a packaged pesto sauce mix saves time in this 20-minute orzo pasta salad recipe.

Ingredients

4 servings

1 cup dried orzo (6 ounces)4 teaspoons packaged pesto sauce mix, such as Knorr brand, divided2 tablespoons olive oil, divided1 pound peeled and deveined fresh or frozen medium shrimp, thawed1 medium zucchini, halved lengthwise and sliced⅛ teaspoon coarse salt⅛ teaspoon freshly cracked pepper1 lemon, halved1 ounce shaved Parmesan cheese

Preparation

Prepare orzo pasta according to package directions. Drain; reserving ¼ cup of the pasta cooking water. Stir 1 teaspoon of the pesto mix into the reserved cooking water; set aside. While pasta is boiling, combine 3 teaspoons of the pesto mix and 1 tablespoon of the olive oil in a large resealable plastic bag. Seal and shake to combine. Add shrimp to bag; seal and turn to coat. Set aside. Cook zucchini in a large skillet in the remaining 1 tablespoon hot oil over medium-high heat for 1 to 2 minutes, stirring often. Add the pesto-marinated shrimp to the skillet and cook for 4 to 5 minutes or until shrimp is opaque. Add the cooked pasta to the skillet with the zucchini and shrimp mixture. Stir in the reserved pasta water until absorbed, scraping up any seasoning in the bottom of the pan. Season with salt and pepper. Squeeze the lemon halves over the pasta just before serving. Top with Parmesan.

DAY 7

Honey Mustard Salmon with Mango Quinoa

In this 30-minute dinner recipe, grilled, honey mustard-coated salmon is served with a tasty grain salad made with quinoa, mango, jalapeño and almonds.

Ingredients

2 servings

1 (8 ounce) fresh or frozen skinless salmon fillet2 teaspoons honey2 teaspoons spicy brown mustard1 large clove garlic, minced⅔ cup cooked quinoa, room temperature½ cup chopped fresh or frozen mango, thawed if frozen1 to 2 tablespoons seeded and finely chopped fresh jalapeño chile pepper (see Tip)1 tablespoon sliced almonds, toasted (see Tip)1 teaspoon olive oil⅛ teaspoon saltPinch ground black pepper2 tablespoons chopped fresh cilantro

Preparation

Thaw salmon, if frozen. Rinse fish and pat dry with paper towels. In a small bowl, stir together honey, mustard and garlic. Brush both sides of salmon with honey mixture. For a gas or charcoal grill, place salmon on grill rack directly over medium heat. Cover and grill for 4 to 6 minutes per ½-inch thickness of fish until salmon begins to flake when tested with a fork, turning once. Meanwhile, in a medium bowl, stir together quinoa, mango, jalapeño pepper, almonds, olive oil, salt and black pepper. Top with fresh cilantro. Serve salmon with quinoa.

Tips: Because chile peppers contain volatile oils that can burn your skin and eyes, avoid direct contact with them as much as possible. When working with chile peppers, wear plastic or rubber gloves. If your bare hands do touch the peppers, wash your hands and nails well with soap and warm water.

To toast nuts, spread in a shallow baking pan lined with parchment paper. Bake in a 350°F oven for 5 to 10 minutes or until golden, shaking pan once or twice.

WEEK 2

DAY 1

Pork Tenderloin with Apple-Onion Chutney

If you'd like the chutney in this pork tenderloin recipe to be both sweet and tart, opt for sweet apples like red or golden delicious and sweet onion.

Ingredients

2 servings

1 (8 ounce) piece pork tenderloin⅛ teaspoon dried thyme, crushed⅛- ¼ teaspoon pepper¾ cup thinly sliced onion8 ounces apples, cored and sliced¼ cup water2 tablespoons cider vinegar1 teaspoon honey¼ teaspoon salt⅛ teaspoon ground cumin (optional)Chopped fresh thyme (optional)

Preparation

Trim fat from pork. Cut the meat in half crosswise. Place each piece, cut side down, between two pieces of plastic wrap. Working from center to edges, pound lightly with the flat side of a meat mallet to ½-inch thickness. Remove the plastic wrap. Sprinkle the meat with dried thyme and pepper. Lightly coat an unheated large skillet with cooking spray. Add the pork. Cook over medium-high heat for 6 to 9 minutes or until a thermometer inserted in the pork registers 145°F, turning once halfway through cooking. Transfer the pork to a plate. Cover and keep warm. For chutney, cook onion in the same skillet about 4 minutes or until tender, stirring occasionally. Stir in apple slices, the water, vinegar, honey, salt, and cumin (if desired). Bring to boiling; reduce heat. Simmer, uncovered, for 4 to 5 minutes or until the liquid is almost evaporated and the apples are tender, stirring occasionally. Return the pork to the skillet and heat through. Divide the pork and chutney between two plates. If desired, garnish with fresh thyme.

DAY 2

Easy Pea & Spinach Carbonara

Fresh pasta cooks up faster than dried, making it a must-have for fast weeknight dinners like this luscious yet healthy meal. Eggs are the base of the creamy sauce. They don't get fully cooked, so use pasteurized-in-the-shell eggs if you prefer.

Ingredients

4 servings

1½ tablespoons extra-virgin olive oil½ cup panko breadcrumbs, preferably whole-wheat1 small clove garlic, minced8 tablespoons grated Parmesan cheese, divided3 tablespoons finely chopped fresh parsley3 large egg yolks1 large egg½ teaspoon ground pepper¼ teaspoon salt1 (9 ounce) package fresh tagliatelle or linguine8 cups baby spinach1 cup peas (fresh or frozen)

Preparation

Put 10 cups of water in a large pot and bring to a boil over high heat. Meanwhile, heat oil in a large skillet over medium-high heat. Add breadcrumbs and garlic; cook, stirring frequently, until toasted, about 2 minutes. Transfer to a small bowl and stir in 2 tablespoons Parmesan and parsley. Set aside. Whisk the remaining 6 tablespoons Parmesan, egg yolks, egg, pepper and salt in a medium bowl. Cook pasta in the boiling water, stirring occasionally, for 1 minute. Add spinach and peas and cook until the pasta is tender, about 1 minute more. Reserve ¼ cup of the cooking water. Drain and place in a large bowl. Slowly whisk the reserved cooking water into the egg mixture. Gradually add the mixture to the pasta, tossing with tongs to combine. Serve topped with the reserved breadcrumb mixture.

DAY 3

Hearty Tomato Soup with Beans & Greens

Garlicky kale and creamy white beans elevate simple canned tomato soup into a 10-minute lunch or dinner that really satisfies. Use a soup with tomato pieces for a heartier texture. Look for a brand that's low- or reduced-sodium, with no more than 450 mg sodium per serving

Ingredients

4 servings

2 (14 ounce) cans low-sodium hearty-style tomato soup1 tablespoon olive oil3 cups chopped kale1 teaspoon minced garlic⅛ teaspoon crushed red pepper (optional)1 (14 ounce) can no-salt-added cannellini beans, rinsed¼ cup grated Parmesan cheese

Preparation

Heat soup in a medium saucepan according to package directions; simmer over low heat as you prepare kale. Heat oil in a large skillet over medium heat. Add kale and cook, stirring, until wilted, 1 to 2 minutes. Stir in garlic and crushed red pepper (if using) and cook for 30 seconds. Stir the greens and beans into the soup and simmer until the beans are heated through, 2 to 3 minutes. Divide the soup among 4 bowls. Serve topped with Parmesan.

DAY 4

Curried Chickpea Stew

Who says a meatless meal isn't filling? Packed with fiber-rich vegetables and chickpeas, this fragrant stew satisfies.

Ingredients

8 servings

1 (10 ounce) bag prewashed spinach or other sturdy greens1½ tablespoons canola oil1 large onion, chopped1 (2 inch) piece fresh ginger, peeled and minced½-1 small jalapeño pepper, seeded and finely chopped3 cloves garlic, minced1 tablespoon curry powder3 medium carrots, peeled and thinly sliced½ medium head cauliflower, broken into bite-size florets (3 cups)2 (15 ounce) cans low-sodium chickpeas, rinsed2 (14 ounce) cans no-salt-added diced tomatoes, drained½ cup fat-free half-and-half⅓ cup "lite" coconut milk

Preparation

Place spinach (or other greens) in a microwave-safe dish; add 1 Tbsp. water and cover. Microwave on High, stirring occasionally, until just wilted, 1 to 2 minutes. Transfer to a colander to drain. When cool enough to handle, squeeze out any excess water. Coarsely chop and set aside. Heat oil in a large nonstick skillet with high sides or a Dutch oven. Add onion and cook, stirring, until translucent, about 8 minutes. Add ginger, jalapeño, garlic, and curry powder; cook, stirring, for 30 seconds. Add carrots and 2 Tbsp. water; cover and cook, stirring occasionally, until the carrots have softened, about 10 minutes (add more water if the mixture becomes dry). Add cauliflower; cover and cook, stirring occasionally, until barely tender-crisp, 5 to 10 minutes more. Stir in chickpeas, tomatoes, half-and-half, and coconut milk. Bring to just below boiling. Reduce heat to low and simmer uncovered, stirring occasionally, for 15 minutes. Stir in the reserved spinach (or greens) and heat through. Transfer half of the mixture (about 5 cups) to a 1½-qt. freezer container; label and freeze for up to 1 month. Serve the remaining half at once, or refrigerate for up to 3 days.

To make ahead: This double-batch recipe makes one meal for tonight (or to refrigerate for up to 3 days) and one to freeze for up to 1 month (see Step 4). To cook from frozen: Thaw overnight in the refrigerator, then microwave on High until heated through, 4 to 5 minutes. You can also reheat the stew in a saucepan until bubbling; add a little water, if needed, to prevent sticking.

DAY 5

Pork & Green Chile Stew

Let your slow cooker work—while you're at work!—and come home to a delicious bowl of hearty stew for dinner. Full of potatoes, hominy, green chiles, and chunks of pork sirloin, this filling stew recipe takes just 25 minutes to prepare in the morning.

Ingredients

6 servings

2 pounds boneless pork sirloin roast or shoulder roast1 tablespoon vegetable oil½ cup chopped onion (1 medium)4 cups peeled and cubed potatoes (4 medium)3 cups water1 (15 ounce) can hominy or whole-kernel corn, drained2 (4 ounce)

cans diced green chile peppers, undrained2 tablespoons quick-cooking tapioca1 teaspoon garlic salt½ teaspoon ground cumin½ teaspoon ancho chile powder½ teaspoon ground pepper¼ teaspoon dried oregano, crushedChopped fresh cilantro (optional)

Preparation

Trim fat from meat. Cut the meat into ½-inch pieces. Cook half of the meat in a large skillet in hot oil over medium-high heat until browned. Using a slotted spoon, remove the meat from the skillet. Repeat with the remaining meat and the onion. Drain off fat. Transfer all of the meat and the onion to a 3½- to 4½-quart slow cooker. Stir in potatoes, the water, hominy, green chile peppers, tapioca, garlic salt, cumin, ancho chile powder, ground pepper, and oregano. Cover and cook on Low for 7 to 8 hours or on High for 4 to 5 hours. If desired, garnish each serving with cilantro.

Equipment: 3½- to 4½-quart slow cooker

DAY 6

Trapanese Pesto Pasta & Zoodles with Salmon

Trapanese pesto is the Sicilian version of the sauce that uses tomatoes and almonds instead of pine nuts. This savory pesto sauce coats low-carb zucchini noodles and heart-healthy seared salmon to create an absolutely delicious pasta dinner.

Ingredients

6 servings

2 zucchini (1¾ lbs. total)1 teaspoon salt, divided½ cup raw whole almonds, toasted1 pound grape tomatoes (3 cups)1 cup packed fresh basil leaves plus ¼ cup chopped, divided2-4 cloves garlic¼ teaspoon crushed red pepper3 tablespoons olive oil, divided8 ounces whole-wheat spaghetti1 pound skinless salmon fillets (about 4 fillets), patted dry¼ teaspoon ground pepper, plus more for garnish2 tablespoons grated Parmesan cheese (optional)

Preparation

Bring a large pot of water to a boil. Cut zucchini into long thin strips with a spiralizer or vegetable peeler. Place in a colander set over a large bowl. Toss with ¼ tsp. salt and let drain for 15 to 20 minutes. Meanwhile, pulse almonds in a food processor until coarsely chopped. Add tomatoes, 1 cup basil leaves, garlic, and crushed red pepper; pulse until coarsely chopped. Add 2 Tbsp. oil and ½ tsp. salt and pulse until combined; set aside. Cook spaghetti in the boiling water according to package directions. Drain and transfer to a large bowl. Gently squeeze the zucchini to remove excess water; add to the bowl with the spaghetti. Heat the remaining 1 Tbsp. oil in a large skillet over medium-high heat until shimmering. Season salmon with pepper and the remaining ¼ tsp. salt. Add the salmon to the pan; cook until the underside is golden and crispy, about 4 minutes. Flip the salmon and cook until it flakes when nudged with a fork, 2 to 4 minutes more. Transfer to a plate and use a fork to gently flake it apart. Add the pesto to the spaghetti mixture; toss to coat. Gently stir in the salmon. Top with the remaining ¼ cup chopped fresh basil. Garnish with Parmesan and additional pepper, if desired.

DAY 7

Jerk Chicken & Pineapple Slaw

Ready in under 30 minutes, this spicy chicken dish with sweet pinapple slaw is perfect for any night of the week.

Ingredients

4 servings

3 heads baby bok choy, trimmed and thinly sliced2 cups shredded red cabbage½ of a fresh pineapple, peeled, cored and chopped2 tablespoons cider vinegar4 teaspoons packed brown sugar2 teaspoons all-purpose flour2 teaspoons jerk seasoning4 skinless, boneless chicken breast halves (1 to 1¼ pounds total)

Preparation

For pineapple slaw, in a very large bowl combine bok choy, cabbage and pineapple. In a small bowl combine cider vinegar and 2 teaspoons of the brown sugar. Drizzle over bok choy mixture; toss to coat. Set aside. In a large resealable plastic bag combine the remaining 2 teaspoons brown sugar, the flour and jerk seasoning. Add chicken; shake well to coat. Grease a grill pan or a heavy 12-inch skillet. Add chicken;

cook over medium heat for 8 to 12 minutes or until no longer pink (170°F), turning once halfway through cooking time. Transfer chicken to a cutting board. Slice chicken and serve with pineapple slaw.

WEEK 3

DAY 1

Jambalaya Stuffed Peppers

In this healthy stuffed peppers recipe, a delicious jambalaya filling of chicken and Cajun spices gets baked inside of bell peppers. Traditional jambalaya is made with green bell peppers, but you can use green, yellow, or orange peppers (or a mix) for this dish. Look for bell peppers with even bottoms, so that they stand upright on their own.

Ingredients

6 servings

6 large green, yellow, or orange bell peppers1½ pounds boneless, skinless chicken thighs, trimmed and cut into 1-inch pieces2 tablespoons salt-free Cajun seasoning (see Tip), divided2 tablespoons olive oil, divided1 link andouille sausage (3-4 oz.), sliced½ cup diced celery1 small onion, diced (½ cup)2 cloves garlic, minced½ teaspoon salt1 (14 ounce) can diced tomatoes¼ cup tomato paste1 cup low-sodium chicken broth1 cup uncooked instant brown rice

Preparation

Preheat oven to 400°F. Line a large rimmed baking sheet with parchment paper or foil. Cut tops off peppers and carefully remove the core and seeds, taking care not to split the skin. Dice the pepper tops and set aside. Place the peppers on the prepared baking sheet; bake for 20 minutes. Remove from oven and let cool. Discard any accumulated liquid in the bottom of the peppers. Meanwhile, season chicken on all sides with 1 Tbsp. Cajun seasoning. Heat 1 Tbsp. oil in a large skillet over medium heat. Add half of the chicken and cook, turning to brown all sides, 4 to 6 minutes. Transfer the chicken to a medium bowl with a slotted spoon. Repeat with the remaining 1 Tbsp. olive oil and the remaining chicken. Add sausage to the now-empty skillet and cook, stirring occasionally, until lightly browned, 1 to 2 minutes. Add celery, onion, and the reserved diced pepper; cook, stirring often, until the onions are translucent, 3 to 5 minutes. Add garlic, the remaining 1 Tbsp. Cajun seasoning, and salt; cook, stirring, for 30 seconds. Add tomatoes and tomato paste; stir to combine, scraping any brown bits off the bottom of the pan. Add broth, rice, and the chicken with any accumulated juices; stir to combine. Bring to a boil. Reduce heat to maintain a simmer and cook, stirring occasionally, until the chicken has cooked through and the rice has softened, 5 to 10 minutes. Remove from heat and stir. Let stand, covered, until all liquid is absorbed, about 10 minutes. Divide the chicken mixture among the peppers, spooning about 1¼ cups into each one and mounding it on top, if necessary. Bake until heated through, about 20 minutes.

Tip: We prefer homemade Cajun seasoning, because it has more flavor and fewer preservatives than the store-bought versions. For salt-free Cajun seasoning, mix 1 Tbsp. paprika, 1 tsp. each onion powder and garlic powder, ½ tsp. each dried oregano and thyme, and ¼ tsp. each cayenne and ground pepper. You will have slightly more than you need for this recipe; use it to season eggs, chicken, fish, or vegetables. (Want to have extra on hand? Multiply these amounts by four.) Store in a covered jar for up to 6 months.

DAY 2

Spinach, Apple & Chicken Salad with Poppy Seed Dressing & Cheese Crisps

Ingredients (4 servings)

3 9-by-14-inch phyllo pastry sheets, thawed4 teaspoons extra-virgin olive oil plus 2 tablespoons, divided1 large egg white, beaten⅓ cup freshly grated Parmigiano-Reggiano cheese1 tablespoon fresh thyme leaves3 tablespoons buttermilk2

tablespoons honey1 tablespoon cider vinegar1 teaspoon poppy seeds½ teaspoon Dijon mustard½ teaspoon kosher salt5 cups baby spinach1½ cups shredded cooked chicken breast1 medium Gala apple, sliced

Preparation

Preheat oven to 350°F. Line a baking sheet with parchment paper. Place 1 sheet of phyllo on the prepared baking sheet. Brush with 2 teaspoons oil. Top with a second sheet of phyllo, pressing gently to adhere. Brush with 2 teaspoons oil. Place the third sheet on top and brush with egg white. Sprinkle with cheese and thyme. Using a pizza cutter or sharp knife, cut the phyllo stack into approximately 2-inch squares. Bake until golden brown, about 8 minutes. Let cool for about 3 minutes. Meanwhile, whisk the remaining 2 tablespoons oil, buttermilk, honey, vinegar, poppy seeds, mustard and salt in a medium bowl. Add spinach, chicken and apple to the bowl and toss to coat. Serve with the phyllo crisps.

To make ahead: Refrigerate dressing (Step 3) for up to 2 days.

Equipment: Parchment paper

DAY 3

Hazelnut-Parsley Roast Tilapia

Sweet and crunchy hazelnuts team up with bright lemon and fresh parsley to add oomph to the tilapia for an easy seafood recipe. Serve this atop a salad or alongside brown rice or orzo.

Ingredients4 servings

2 tablespoons olive oil, divided4 (5 ounce) tilapia fillets (fresh or frozen, thawed)⅓ cup finely chopped hazelnuts¼ cup finely chopped fresh parsley1 small shallot, minced2 teaspoons lemon zest⅛ teaspoon salt plus ¼ teaspoon, divided¼ teaspoon ground pepper, divided1½ tablespoons lemon juice

Preparation

Preheat oven to 450°F. Line a large rimmed baking sheet with foil; brush with 1 Tbsp. oil. Bring fish to room temperature by letting it stand on the counter for 15 minutes. Meanwhile, stir together hazelnuts, parsley, shallot, lemon zest, 1 tsp. oil, ⅛ tsp. salt, and ⅛ tsp. pepper in a small bowl. Pat both sides of the fish dry with a paper towel. Place the fish on the prepared baking sheet. Brush both sides of the fish with lemon juice and the remaining 2 tsp. oil. Season both sides evenly with the remaining ¼ tsp. salt and ⅛ tsp. pepper. Divide the hazelnut mixture evenly among the tops of the fillets and pat gently to adhere. Roast the fish until it is opaque, firm, and just beginning to flake, 7 to 10 minutes. Serve immediately.

DAY 4

Charred Vegetable & Bean Tostadas with

Pile vegetables and black beans onto crisp tostadas and top them off with lime crema for a vegetarian dinner the whole family will love. Charring the vegetables under the broiler infuses them with smoky flavor while cooking them quickly.

.Ingredients 6 servings

Lime Crema5 tablespoons sour cream⅛ teaspoon lime zest2 teaspoons lime juice⅛ teaspoon kosher saltTostadas6 corn tortillas2 tablespoons canola oil plus 2 teaspoons, divided4 cloves garlic, sliced, divided1½ teaspoons ground cumin1 teaspoon kosher salt, divided⅛ teaspoon chipotle chile powder2 (15 ounce) cans no-salt-added black beans, rinsed¼ cup water, plus more as needed2 medium red bell peppers, sliced1 large red onion, halved and sliced2 medium zucchini, halved and sliced ½ inch thick1 cup fresh or frozen corn kernels¼ teaspoon ground pepper1 cup thinly shredded cabbage¼ cup chopped fresh cilantro6 tablespoons crumbled cotija cheese

Preparation

To prepare crema: Combine sour cream, lime zest, lime juice and salt in a small bowl. Set aside. To prepare tostadas: Position a rack in upper third of oven; preheat to 400°F. Brush both sides of tortillas with 1 tablespoon oil and arrange on a baking sheet. (It's OK if they overlap a bit; they will shrink as they cook.) Bake, turning once halfway, until browned and crisp, about 10 minutes. Transfer to a wire rack and let cool. Meanwhile, heat 2 teaspoons oil in a large skillet over medium heat. Add 1 garlic clove and cook, stirring occasionally, until fragrant, about 30 seconds. Add cumin, ½ teaspoon salt and chile powder; cook, stirring, for 30 seconds more. Add beans and cook, stirring occasionally, until heated through, about 4 minutes. Transfer the beans to a food processor and add ¼ cup water. Pulse until smooth, adding more water, 1 tablespoon at a time, if needed. Preheat broiler to high. Toss bell peppers, onion, zucchini, corn, ground pepper, the remaining 3 garlic cloves, 1 tablespoon oil and ½ teaspoon salt in a large bowl. Spread on a large rimmed baking sheet. Broil, stirring occasionally, until lightly charred, 8 to 12 minutes. Top the tostadas with some of the beans, charred vegetables, cabbage, cilantro, cheese and the reserved crema.

DAY 5

Pistachio-Crusted Baked Trout

Finely chopped pistachios take center stage in this baked fish recipe. Toasted seeds are mixed with the pistachios to create a fragrant and crunchy crust which nicely compliments the tender fish.

Ingredients4 servings

4 (4-5 ounce) fresh or frozen trout fillets (see Tip)½ teaspoon coriander seeds½ teaspoon cumin seeds½ teaspoon caraway seeds4 teaspoons olive oil1 teaspoon finely shredded lemon peel1 clove garlic, minced½ teaspoon kosher salt¼ teaspoon ground cinnamon¼ teaspoon ground pepper¼ cup pistachio nuts, finely chopped4 lemon wedges

Preparation

Thaw fish, if frozen. Preheat oven to 350°F. Line a shallow baking pan with foil and coat with cooking spray; set aside. Heat a small saucepan over low heat; add coriander seeds, cumin seeds, and caraway seeds. Cook and stir for 4 minutes or until fragrant and golden. (Do not allow the seeds to burn or they will taste bitter.) Remove from heat. Using a small food processor or a mortar and pestle, grind the seeds. Stir in oil, lemon peel, garlic, salt, cinnamon, and pepper. Place pistachios in a small bowl; set aside. Rinse the fish; pat dry with paper towels. Spread one side of the fish fillets with the spice mixture. Bringing up two opposite ends, fold the fish into thirds. Dip the top and the sides of the fish bundles into the nuts to coat; place in the prepared baking pan. Sprinkle with any remaining nuts. Bake for 15 to 20 minutes or until the fish begins to flake when tested with a fork (145°F). Serve with lemon wedges.

Tip: Save some time by asking your butcher or fishmonger to fillet the fish and remove the skin.

DAY 6

Pork Medallions with Cranberry-Onion Relish

Pork tenderloin is a great choice for dinner when it's thinly sliced into quick-cooking medallions. A tart cranberry and onion relish adds delicious taste to each bite of this 30-minute entree.

Ingredients

4 servings

12 ounces pork tenderloin¼ cup all-purpose flourPinch of saltPinch of ground pepper2 tablespoons olive oil, divided1 small onion, thinly sliced¼ cup dried cranberries¼ cup reduced-sodium chicken broth1 tablespoon balsamic vinegar

Preparation

Trim fat from pork. Cut the pork crosswise into eight slices. Place each slice between two pieces of plastic wrap. Using the flat side of a meat mallet, lightly pound the pork to ¼-inch thickness. Discard plastic wrap. Combine flour, salt, and pepper in a shallow dish. Dip the pork slices into the flour mixture, turning to coat. Coat a heavy large skillet with cooking spray. Add 1 tablespoon oil to the skillet; heat over medium-high heat. Add four pork slices to the hot oil; cook for 3 to 4 minutes or until the pork is slightly pink in the center, turning once halfway through the cooking time. Transfer the pork to a serving platter; cover with foil to keep warm. Repeat with the remaining 1 tablespoon oil and the remaining four pork slices. Cook onion in the same skillet over medium heat for about 4 minutes or until crisp-tender. Combine cranberries, broth, and vinegar in a small bowl; carefully add to the skillet. Heat through. Serve the onion mixture over the pork slices.

DAY 7

Lemon Chicken & Rice

This easy Persian-inspired chicken and rice dish has a beautiful golden color and a wonderful fragrance. If you have saffron in the cupboard, do add that optional pinch; just a little will enhance the flavor and aroma of the dish.

Ingredients

8 servings

2 tablespoons olive oil, divided8 boneless, skinless chicken thighs (1¼-1½ lbs. total), trimmed2 large onions, thinly sliced½ teaspoon salt, divided3 cloves garlic, minced2 teaspoons ground turmeric1 teaspoon paprikaGenerous pinch of saffron (optional)3 cups shredded cabbage (about ½ small head)4 cups cooked brown rice, preferably basmati or jasmine¼ cup lemon juice2 tablespoons chopped fresh Italian parsley (optional)1 lemon, sliced (optional)

Preparation

Prep

50 m

Ready In

1 h 35 m

Preheat oven to 375°F. Coat two 8-inch-square baking dishes or foil pans with cooking spray (see Tip). Heat 1 Tbsp. oil in a large nonstick skillet over medium-high heat. Add 4 chicken thighs, and cook, turning once, until both sides are lightly browned, about 4 minutes. Transfer the chicken to a plate and set aside. Repeat with the remaining chicken thighs. Pour off all but about 1 Tbsp. fat from the pan. Add the remaining 1 Tbsp. oil and onions to the pan and sprinkle with ¼ tsp. salt. Cook, stirring, until soft and golden, 12 to 15 minutes. Stir in garlic, turmeric, paprika, and saffron, if using; cook, stirring, for 2 minutes. Transfer the onions to a plate and set aside. Return the pan to medium-high heat and add cabbage. Cook, stirring, until wilted, about 3 minutes. Stir in rice, lemon juice, the remaining ¼ tsp. salt, and half of the reserved onion. Continue cooking until the rice is well coated and heated through, 5 to 7 minutes. Divide the rice mixture between the prepared baking dishes; nestle 4 of the reserved chicken thighs in each dish. Top each with half of the remaining cooked onions. Cover both dishes with foil. Label one and freeze for up to 1 month. Bake the remaining casserole, covered, for 30 minutes. Uncover and continue baking until a thermometer inserted in the thickest part of the chicken registers 165°F and the onions are starting to brown around the edges, 5 to 10 minutes more. Garnish with parsley and lemon slices, if desired.

Tip: Instead of freezing half, you can bake the full recipe in a 9x13-inch baking pan. In Step 6, bake, covered, for an additional 10 minutes.

To make ahead: This double-batch recipe makes one meal for tonight and one to freeze for up to 1 month (see Step 5). To cook from frozen: Thaw overnight in the refrigerator, then bake as directed in Steps 6-7, adding an additional 10 minutes baking time once uncovered.

Equipment: Two 8-inch-square baking dishes or foil pans

WEEK 4

DAY 1

Pumpkin Seed Salmon with Maple-Spice

Because this one-pan meal is ready in just 35 minutes, it's a good choice for a healthy recipe after you've had a long day at the office. Maple-spiced carrots cook alongside pepita-crusted salmon fillets and deliver amazing taste and nutrition in a dinner the whole family will devour.

Ingredients

4 servings

4 (4-5 ounce) fresh or frozen salmon fillets1 pound carrots, cut diagonally into ¼-inch slices¼ cup pure maple syrup, divided½ teaspoon salt, divided½ teaspoon pumpkin pie spice8 multi-grain saltine crackers, finely crushed3 tablespoons finely chopped salted, roasted pumpkin seeds (pepitas) plus 2 teaspoons, dividedCooking spray

Preparation

Thaw fish, if frozen. Preheat oven to 425°F. Line a 15x10-inch baking pan with foil; set aside. Combine carrots, 3 tablespoons maple syrup, ¼ teaspoon salt, and the pumpkin pie spice in a large bowl. Arrange the carrots on one-half of the prepared baking pan. Bake for 10 minutes. Meanwhile, rinse the fish; pat dry with paper towels. Combine crushed crackers, 3 tablespoons of the pumpkin seeds, and the remaining ¼ teaspoon salt in a shallow dish. Brush the top of the fish with the remaining 1 tablespoon maple syrup. Sprinkle with the cracker mixture, pressing to adhere. Place the fish in the baking pan next to the carrots. Lightly coat the top of the fish with cooking spray. Bake for 10 to 15 minutes more or until the fish flakes easily when tested with a fork and the carrots are tender. To serve, divide the carrots among dinner plates and sprinkle with the remaining 2 teaspoons pumpkin seeds. Top with the salmon.

Salmon Couscous Salad

This healthy and easy salad is designed to be made with precooked or leftover salmon. To quickly cook salmon, lightly brush with olive oil, then roast in a 450°F oven until the fish is opaque and firm, 8 to 12 minutes.

Ingredients

1 serving

¼ cup sliced cremini mushrooms¼ cup diced eggplant3 cups baby spinach2 tablespoons white-wine vinaigrette, divided (see Tip)¼ cup cooked Israeli couscous, preferably whole-wheat4 ounces cooked salmon¼ cup sliced dried apricots2 tablespoons crumbled goat cheese (½ ounce)

Preparation

Coat a small skillet with cooking spray and heat over medium-high heat. Add mushrooms and eggplant; cook, stirring, until lightly browned and juices have been released, 3 to 5 minutes. Remove from heat and set aside. Toss spinach with 1 Tbsp. plus 1 tsp. vinaigrette and place on a 9-inch plate. Toss couscous with the remaining 2 tsp. vinaigrette and place on top of the spinach. Place salmon on top. Top with the cooked vegetables, dried apricots, and goat cheese.

Tip: To make a quick white-wine vinaigrette, whisk 2 Tbsp. white-wine vinegar with ⅛ tsp. each salt and pepper. Slowly whisk in ¼ cup extra-virgin olive oil until blended. Extra dressing will keep, covered, in the refrigerator for up to 5 days. Bring to room temperature before using.

DAY 2

Vegan Cauliflower Fettuccine Alfredo with Kale

Ingredients

6 servings

½ cup fresh whole-wheat breadcrumbs, toasted1 tablespoon chopped fresh parsley½ teaspoon grated lemon zest4 cups cauliflower florets (1 small head)1 cup raw cashews8 ounces whole-wheat fettuccine4 cups lightly packed thinly sliced kale3 tablespoons lemon juice2 tablespoons white miso2 teaspoons garlic powder2 teaspoons onion powder¾ teaspoon salt1 cup water

Preparation

Put a large pot of water on to boil. Combine breadcrumbs, parsley and lemon zest in a small bowl. Set aside. Add cauliflower and cashews to the boiling water; cook until the cauliflower is very tender, about 15 minutes. Using a slotted spoon, transfer cauliflower and cashews to a blender. Add pasta to the boiling water and cook, stirring occasionally, for 10 minutes. Add kale and cook until the pasta is just tender, about 1 minute more. Drain; return the pasta and kale to the pot. Add lemon juice, miso, garlic powder, onion powder, salt and 1 cup water to the blender; process until smooth. Add the sauce to the pasta and stir until well coated. Serve topped with the breadcrumb mixture.

DAY 3

Curried Sweet Potato & Peanut Soup
In this flavorful soup recipe, sweet potatoes simmer in a quick coconut curry, resulting in a creamy, thick broth punctuated by notes of garlic and ginger. We love peanuts for their inexpensive price and versatile flavor. They're also a great source of protein—1 ounce has 7 grams.

Ingredients

6 servings

2 tablespoons canola oil1½ cups diced yellow onion1 tablespoon minced garlic1 tablespoon minced fresh ginger4 teaspoons red curry paste (see Tip)1 serrano chile, ribs and seeds removed, minced1 pound sweet potatoes, peeled and cubed (½-inch pieces)3 cups water1 cup "lite" coconut milk¾ cup unsalted dry-roasted peanuts1 (15 ounce) can white beans, rinsed¾ teaspoon salt¼ teaspoon ground pepper¼ cup chopped fresh cilantro2 tablespoons lime juice¼ cup unsalted roasted pumpkin seedsLime wedges

Preparation

Heat oil in a large pot over medium-high heat. Add onion and cook, stirring often, until softened and translucent, about 4 minutes. Stir in garlic, ginger, curry paste, and serrano; cook, stirring, for 1 minute. Stir in sweet potatoes and water; bring to a boil. Reduce heat to medium-low and simmer, partially covered, until the sweet potatoes are soft, 10 to 12 minutes. Transfer half of the soup to a blender, along with coconut milk and peanuts; puree. (Use caution when pureeing hot liquids.) Return to the pot with the remaining soup. Stir in beans, salt, and pepper; heat through. Remove from the heat. Stir in cilantro and lime juice. Serve with pumpkin seeds and lime wedges.

Tip: You can find red curry paste in the Asian section of many grocery stores, packaged in a small glass jar.

To make ahead: Refrigerate soup for up to 3 days. Reheat before serving.

DAY 4

Spinach & Strawberry Salad with Poppy Seed Dressing

Homemade poppy seed dressing pairs beautifully with tender spinach, crunchy almonds and juicy berries for a fantastically refreshing and easy spring salad. To make ahead, whisk dressing, combine salad ingredients and store separately. Toss the salad with the dressing just before serving. To make it a complete meal, top with grilled chicken or shrimp.

Ingredients

4 servings

2½ tablespoons mayonnaise1½ tablespoons cider vinegar1 tablespoon extra-virgin olive oil1 teaspoon poppy seeds1 teaspoon sugar¼ teaspoon salt¼ teaspoon ground pepper1 (5 ounce) package baby spinach1 cup sliced strawberries¼ cup toasted sliced almonds

Preparation

Whisk mayonnaise, vinegar, oil, poppy seeds, sugar, salt and pepper in a large bowl. Add spinach and strawberries and toss to coat. Sprinkle with almonds.

DAY 5

Slow-Cooked Pork Tacos with Chipotle Aioli

Follow this pork taco recipe as is to serve four and you'll have enough shredded pork leftover to make it again next week. It's so good, however, that we recommend doubling the rest of the ingredients and inviting over four more friends to enjoy everything right away!

Ingredients

4 servings

1 (2 to 2½ pound) boneless pork sirloin roast3 tablespoons reduced-sodium taco seasoning mix1 (14.5 ounce) can no-salt-added diced tomatoes, undrained1 cup shredded romaine lettuce1 cup chopped mango⅔ cup thin bite-size strips, peeled jicama½ cup light mayonnaise2 tablespoons lime juice2 cloves garlic, minced½ to 1 teaspoon finely chopped canned chipotle pepper in adobo sauce (see Tip)8 (6 inch) corn tortillas, warmed¼ cup coarsely chopped fresh cilantro

Preparation

Prep

40 m

Ready In

4 h 10 m

Trim fat from roast. Sprinkle with taco seasoning mix; rub in with your fingers. Place the roast in a 3½- or 4-quart slow cooker. Add undrained tomatoes; cover and cook on Low for 7 to 8 hours or on High for 3½ to 4 hours. Remove the roast, reserving cooking liquid. Shred the meat using two forks. Toss the meat with enough cooking liquid to moisten. Set half of the meat aside (about 2½ cups) and place the remainder in an airtight container for later use (see Tip). Combine lettuce, mango, and jicama in a medium bowl. For chipotle aioli, combine mayonnaise, lime juice, garlic, and chipotle pepper in a small bowl. Serve the shredded meat, the lettuce mixture, and the chipotle aioli in tortillas. Sprinkle with cilantro.

Tips: If desired, substitute ¼ teaspoon ground chipotle chile pepper for the canned chipotle pepper.

Leftover shredded meat can be stored in an airtight container in the refrigerator up to 3 days or freezer for up to 3 months.

Equipment: 3½- or 4-quart slow cooker

DAY 6

Tofu & Snow Pea Stir-Fry with Peanut Sauce

A fast dinner recipe perfect for busy weeknights, this easy stir-fry recipe will quickly become a favorite. To save time, use precooked rice or cook rice a day ahead.

Ingredients

4 servings

⅓ cup unsalted natural peanut butter3 tablespoons rice vinegar2 tablespoons low-sodium soy sauce2 teaspoons brown sugar (see Tip)2 teaspoons hot sauce, such as Sriracha1 (14 ounce) package extra-firm or firm tofu (see Tip)4 teaspoons canola oil, divided1 (14 ounce) package frozen (not thawed) pepper stir-fry vegetables2 tablespoons finely chopped or grated fresh ginger3 cloves garlic, minced2 cups fresh snow peas, trimmed2 tablespoons water, plus more if needed4 tablespoons unsalted roasted peanuts2 cups cooked brown rice

Preparation

Prep

30 m

Ready In

30 m

Combine peanut butter, vinegar, soy sauce, sugar, and hot sauce in a medium bowl; whisk until smooth. Set aside. Drain tofu; pat dry with a paper towel. Cut into ¾-inch cubes; pat dry again. Heat 2 tsp. oil in a large nonstick skillet over medium-high heat. Add half the tofu and let cook, undisturbed, until lightly browned underneath, about 2 minutes. Stir and continue cooking, stirring occasionally, until browned all over, 1 to 2 minutes. Transfer to a plate. Add 1 tsp. oil to the pan, then the remaining tofu; repeat. Add the remaining 1 tsp. oil to the pan. Add frozen vegetables, ginger, and garlic; stir-fry until the ginger and garlic are fragrant and the vegetables have thawed, 2 to 3 minutes. Stir in snow peas. Add water, cover and cook until the peas are crisp-tender, 3 to 4 minutes. Push the vegetables to the edges of the pan. Add the reserved peanut sauce to the center and cook, stirring, until hot, about 30 seconds. Stir the vegetables into the sauce. Add the reserved tofu and cook, stirring, until heated through, 30 to 60 seconds. If necessary, add more water to make a creamy sauce. Sprinkle each serving with 1 Tbsp. peanuts; serve with rice.

Tips: If using a sugar substitute, we recommend Splenda Brown Sugar Blend. Follow package directions for 2 tsp. equivalent. Nutrition Per Serving with Substitute: Same as below except CAL 506, CARB 47g (sugars 9g), POTASSIUM 316mg.

Don't like tofu? Substitute 12 oz. boneless, skinless chicken breast or chicken tenders, cut into thin slices. When you brown the chicken in Step 3, be sure that it is cooked through.

DAY 7

Chicken & Sun-Dried Tomato Orzo

Sun-dried tomatoes and Romano cheese pack a flavorful punch along with the tantalizing aroma of fresh marjoram in this rustic Italian-inspired dish. Serve with sautéed fresh spinach or steamed broccolini.

Ingredients 4 servings

8 ounces orzo, preferably whole-wheat1 cup water½ cup chopped sun-dried tomatoes, (not oil-packed), divided1 plum tomato, diced1 clove garlic, peeled3 teaspoons chopped fresh marjoram, divided1 tablespoon red-wine vinegar2 teaspoons plus 1 tablespoon extra-virgin olive oil, divided4 boneless, skinless chicken breasts, trimmed (1-1¼ pounds)¼ teaspoon salt¼ teaspoon freshly ground pepper1 9-ounce package frozen artichoke hearts, thawed½ cup finely shredded Romano cheese, divided

Preparation

Cook orzo in a large saucepan of boiling water until just tender, 8 to 10 minutes or according to package directions. Drain and rinse. Meanwhile, place 1 cup water, ¼ cup sun-dried tomatoes, plum tomato, garlic, 2 teaspoons marjoram, vinegar and 2 teaspoons oil in a blender. Blend until just a few chunks remain. Season chicken with salt and pepper on both sides. Heat remaining 1 tablespoon oil in a large skillet over medium-high heat. Add the chicken and cook, adjusting the heat as necessary to prevent burning, until golden outside and no longer pink in the middle, 3 to 5 minutes per side. Transfer to a plate; tent with foil to keep warm. Pour the tomato sauce into the pan and bring to a boil. Measure out ½ cup sauce to a small bowl. Add the remaining ¼ cup sun-dried tomatoes to the pan along with the orzo, artichoke hearts and 6 tablespoons cheese. Cook, stirring, until heated through, 1 to 2 minutes. Divide among 4 plates. Slice the chicken. Top each portion of pasta with sliced chicken, 2 tablespoons of the reserved tomato sauce and a sprinkling of the remaining cheese and marjoram.

ITS FULLEST

Kidney dialysis diet helps maintain a balance of electrolytes, minerals, and fluids in patients who are on dialysis. The special diet is important because dialysis alone does not effectively remove all waste products. These waste products can also build up between dialysis treatments.

Most dialysis patients urinate very little or not at all, and therefore fluid restriction between treatments is very important.

Without urination, fluid will build up in the body and cause excess fluid in the heart, lungs, and ankles.

The purpose of dialysis is that it removes excess water and nitrogenous wastes, reducing the manifestations of renal failure.

Dialysis can be used temporarily if the client has acute renal failure or as a permanent, lifesustaining treatment if the client had chronic renal failure. In the latter case, the dialysis must continue for the rest of a patient's life unless successful kidney transplantation is performed.

Kidney dialysis diet, coupled with dialysis, is also used to control uremia and to physically prepare the client to receive a transplanted kidney. Dialysis is usually necessary to keep the client alive until a suitable kidney donor kidney is found. If the transplanted kidney does not immediately function adequately, dialysis may help prevent uremia until the kidney begins functioning properly.

Here are some general guidelines on what to do before or after dialysis treatment has started:

✦ Eat regular meals.

- ✦ Include plenty of variety in your diet. This will provide you with essential nutrients such as protein, calories, vitamins, and minerals. These nutrients keep you well nourished.

- ✦ Eat some high-fiber foods such as whole-grain bread and cereals.

- ✦ Eat only moderate amounts of fats.

- ✦ Avoid adding extra salt to foods if you have high blood pressure.

You can say that these guidelines are very practical and easy to follow. But I'm still including it here in this article because you need to be reminded of this fact. Although we know what's necessarily good, we don't always do it. In fact, most of us just do the opposite because we think of ourselves as invincible to the many health risk factors in our environment. But now that you have a renal disease, you need to follow these guidelines more than ever.

Kidney dialysis diet will not focus only on the general guidelines but also on specific measures on what to do pre and post dialysis treatment.

These measures are very important because they can help preserve renal function and delay the need for transplantation as long as possible.

WHY HIGH-PROTEIN DIETS ACCELERATE LOSS OF
KIDNEY FUNCTION

The problem with this dietary nutrient is the manner in which it is metabolized. The enzymes present in the gastrointestinal tract break down proteins into individual amino acids. They are further divided into nitrogen and non-nitrogen parts. The non-nitrogen parts are used by the body for the production of fat or glucose and the generation of energy or are recycled into amino acids. The nitrogenous compounds are waste products and are flushed from the system.

The kidneys take part in numerous body functions primarily waste removal. Healthy excretory organs are able to remove protein wastes even when consumed in large amounts. However, the diminished function, in the case of CKD, leads to the accumulation of non-nitrogenous compounds in the liver and kidneys. The condition is called Blood Urea Nitrogen and it causes dehydration. Thus by eliminating these food types, you can reduce the strain on the renal organs and prolong their life.

Protein Diet for Kidney Disease Patients - Before and During Dialysis

Chronic kidney disease treatment supports a protein-restricted diet. Nonetheless, it cannot be severely restricted because it sustains important body activities. They are nicknamed the "building blocks of life". Amino acids participate in all cell functions. They build muscle mass and help maintain a healthy weight. Some proteins enable body movements while others protect the body from germs. Hence, a renal diet calls for a restriction of this dietary nutrient to a nominal amount per day.

The daily protein intake differs for a CKD patient on dialysis and not on dialysis. A person in the early stages of CKD using medication as a primary treatment must have a low protein diet. The quality and amount of protein vary based on food. Meat, eggs, and milk are rich sources of proteins. They are also high fat and cholesterol foods. Chicken breast, low-fat dairy foods, lean red meats, fish and soy products are kidney-friendly and heart-friendly foods.

On the contrary, persons on dialysis are advised to increase their protein intake. Dialysis is an artificial filtration process used to help the excretory organs wash out wastes from the blood. But while removing wastes, it also removes necessary nutrients.

Therefore, when you start dialysis sessions, you will have to eat more protein. It is safe to eat 810 ounces of protein per day.

Foods you can include in your diet are an egg (egg white or egg white powder), poultry, fish and pork.

When you suffer from CKD or any other ailments, you should not make any dietary changes on your own. Consult a dietician or a nutritionist. A health care professional will guide you on an appropriate eating plan designed to meet your health requirements and in keeping in mind your health condition.

A Chronic Kidney Disease Diet Plan For Diabetics

Out of the total number of people who suffer diabetes in the United States, more than 50% are also diagnosed with decreased renal function. Diabetes is the culprit. Major fluctuations in the blood sugar levels damage blood vessels in the kidneys and reduce their ability to filter the blood properly. The insulin imbalance also affects the nerves that signal when the bladder is full.

Accumulation of urine in the bladder can cause severe urinary tract infections. The infection can spread to other organs if not treated. To add, improper emptying of the bladder has a negative impact on the excretory organs.

Chronic kidney disease and diabetes is a tricky combination because there are diet restrictions for both. You need a diet plan that will strike a balance between the two; one that stabilizes blood sugar levels while simultaneously ensuring a minimum buildup of waste and fluids in the body. Not only this, but it should also be such that it fulfills your nutritional and caloric requirements.

So, what should you eat and what shouldn't you? We'll help you decide.

Dietary Recommendations

If you have both diabetes and kidney disease, you should eat low glycemic foods. Controlling blood glucose levels helps prevent further damage to kidneys. This is more essential if you're currently on hemodialysis. Foods with low glycemic index keep a tab on blood glucose and thereby control thirst and fluid gain.

Proteins, fats, carbohydrates, potassium, phosphorus, and sodium should be consumed in limited quantities. It all depends on your specific health condition. You should decrease the use of salts, salty foods, and salt substitutes. Limiting salt intake decreases the amount of fluid retained by the body. Avoid adding salt to your food when at the dining table. Read food labels carefully and choose lower sodium options. You should cut back your intake of deli-meats, canned foods convenience meals, sauces, coatings, marinades, and toppings as they have large amounts of hidden sodium.

Diet for kidney patients recommends less protein while a diabetic diet focuses on lean protein. The amount of protein you can consume depends on the stage of CKD. Those on dialysis can eat a larger proportion of protein. Protein foods you can eat include lean meats, fish, poultry and skimmed or fat-free milk. Try as much as possible to avoid diet colas, lemonades, and herbal teas as they are rich sources of phosphorus in addition to salt. Diabetes and chronic kidney disease patients can take a moderate amount of complex carbohydrates. Eat fresh fruits and vegetable instead of the canned varieties. Avoid water-rich fruits and vegetables.

Portion Control

Portion control is an important aspect of a diabetic renal diet. You should control the amount of food you eat at every meal. A nutritionist will guide you on appropriate portion sizes and also help you identify portion sizes. Many-a-times what we believe to be one serving (restaurant serving) actually measures as three servings. You can divide the total calorie intake into several smaller meals. Eat meals at regular intervals to maintain blood glucose levels.

This is a basic idea of the foods to eat and avoid if you've been diagnosed with diabetes and CKD. It is advised you work with a dietician to design an eating plan that's right for you. Do not make any changes to your diet without a doctor's knowledge.

Antony Jason Willfour

AN OVERVIEW OF TREATMENT STRATEGIES FOR
RENAL FAILURE

What is Renal Failure

Renal failure is characterized by a loss in kidney function secondary to any number of conditions including diabetes, high blood pressure, congenital abnormalities, drug overdose, medication reactions, and many others. The fact that the kidneys are the primary means by which excess water and waste are filtered from the bloodstream means that a loss in capacity can quickly result in deadly accumulations of particles that harm vital organ systems. Fortunately, there are a couple of treatment options available to kidney failure patients that can dramatically improve their quality of life and increase the number of years they have on Earth. For those who plan to work in the dialysis industry as a technician, it is important to understand how the kidneys function and how dialysis works so that individuals are prepared to help answer any questions or concerns that patients might have.

The kidneys are situated in the lower rear quadrant of the abdominal cavity in front of the lower set of ribs. These anatomical structures are about the size of a fist and they contain a complex network of tubes that are designed to facilitate the filtration of excess water and waste from the blood as well as the absorption of nutrients that are unintentionally filtered.

Included in the body's vascular system are a renal artery and renal vein that are responsible for directing blood to the kidneys and carrying it from the kidneys back to the main circulatory system.

Each time the heart contracts, blood passes through the complex vascular system within the kidneys and is exposed to permeable membranes that contain pores just large

115

enough to allow water and waste particles to pass through. The filtrate is collected by the kidneys and sent to the bladder where it is stored as urine until it can be excreted.

When the kidneys become damaged, they can no longer filter potentially harmful particles from the blood as they could when they were fully functional. If the loss in kidney function exceeds a certain percentage, individuals start to experience uncomfortable signs and symptoms of kidney failure such as water retention, nausea, and skin irritation. At this point, it becomes important to start considering treatment options that can partially compensate for the loss in the body's ability to get rid of molecules that it no longer needs and that could harm important organs. The two most common treatment options for renal failure include a kidney transplant and dialysis therapy. Because spare kidneys can be difficult to find, most patients are dependent on dialysis for survival while they wait for a donor's kidney.

Dialysis is a medical procedure that uses a machine to recreate the filtration mechanism found in a healthy kidney. Prior to beginning the treatment process, a dialysis patient must have a special vascular access point known as a fistula or anastomosis created just under the skin. This access point is used to connect the patient to the tubes that are used to carry blood from the body to the machine and back to the body. During each treatment, the patient sits for many hours as the machine cleans the blood and adds essential nutrients that the patient may be lacking. While the machine does do a decent job of replacing a portion of the filtration capacity of the kidneys, it cannot fully compensate for the loss in function and is dependent on the patient's compliance with a strict renal diet for optimal health outcomes.

Some renal failure patients are eligible for an alternate self-administered form of treatment known as peritoneal dialysis. This approach to cleaning the blood uses the vascular system inside the abdominal cavity to filter excess water and waste. Individuals who qualify for this approach to therapy must have a tube surgically implanted in the abdominal wall so that filtration fluid can be added and removed. The most concerning risk factor associated with this type of dialysis are the possibility of the surgical site becoming infected. If this happens, the patients may suffer from adverse side effects and may be required to return to a clinic for ongoing treatment.

How Renal Diets Can Make A Huge Difference In Your Day To Day Wellness

Renal diets help those suffering from kidney disease to raise their quality of life and how they feel daily.

Certain types of food can be detrimental to diseased kidneys, so make sure to have a good working knowledge of not only the disease but also how it affects your body in particular.

Kidney disease is not something you want, but there are ways of raising your quality of life high by changing your diet. In truth, renal diets help you manage your health and keep your kidney disease reduced.

You need to remember- modifying your diet is not going to heal everyone but it may be able to help everyone. This does not mean that a diet is a cure-all for everybody so do not think of this essay as medical advice rather as more of a guideline.

Your doctor can provide lots more advice than this exposition, and should always be consulted or notified of any change in your condition.

If you have kidney problems renal diets are essential to regulating your health and assisting you in feeling better. There are entire cookbooks devoted to renal diets or you could check with with a registered dietitian for recommendations. If you use a Kindle or iPad, you can even download and view these books instantly.

Dietitians have experience working with those suffering from kidney problems, and can give some general do's and don'ts to follow, such as:

+ Regulate Potassium intake - fruits like strawberries and apples along with vegetables like cauliflower, cabbage and broccoli are low in Potassium.

+ Monitor your Phosphorous intake - Non-dairy creamer, pasta, cereals, and rice are on the OK list.

+ Limit Fluid Intake - forty-eight oz. of fluid per day is the recommended level for renal diets- be sure to count the fluid in items like grapes, ice cream, oranges, et cetera.

+ Monitor your salt intake - You'll need to be a label reader to make sure you keep your salt intake low- know what you are putting into your body and the result it may have.

+ Regulate your intake of protein - maintain 5- 7 ounces. Utilizing egg substitutes instead of regular eggs is a good technique to keep your protein intake low.

Should you choose to utilize a dietitian, they are able to point you precisely to what you should and should not consume and why.

Being aware of the effect food has on your body is powerful information and can help how you feel on a day to day basis.

THE INS AND OUTS OF A HEALTHY RENAL DIET

When it comes to kidney health, diet goes a long way to both protect your kidneys and improve their function if you are suffering from kidney damage. The best renal diet can vary depending upon your level of kidney health, your level of physical activity, and other health conditions that may be present.

While the appropriate renal diet may alter depending on your kidney health there are some simple protocols that you can follow, and nutrients that you should be aware of that may need to be included or avoided in your diet. Nutrition can always be used as a form of medicine and here we will look at the benefits and dangers in several foods and nutrients.

Food And Nutrients In Renal Diet

Protein often causes a sense of confusion when it comes to kidney health and the renal diet. The best option is to talk to your doctor regarding protein requirements as they vary according to your physical activity levels, but basically speaking if you have kidney damage you need to limit your protein intake. However, of course, we do need some protein in our diet so it comes down to choices. It is recommended to cut out dairy and red meat sources of protein, as they are often high in saturated fats and sometimes sodium, which places an excess burden upon both the kidneys and cardiovascular system.

Chicken is preferable to red meat, however, it is often pumped full of hormones, so organic varieties are always preferable. Fish, however, is an excellent source of protein as it is high in essential fatty acids, which are fantastic for many aspects of health and have a strong antiinflammatory action, which is beneficial for the kidneys. Soy proteins such as tofu and tempeh are also recommended, and when eaten regularly they have actually shown to help slow the progression of kidney damage.

There are three dietary minerals that need to be avoided as part of the renal diet. This is because the kidneys need to filter the blood of these minerals to achieve the correct levels, but in kidney damage, this does not occur effectively and levels can build up in the blood and become dangerous. In particular, we are referring to phosphorus, potassium, and sodium, and we will look at why each of these is a problem and the foods that should be avoided.

On the other hand, not only the renal diet but all diets should avoid high levels of sodium. Sodium can increase blood pressure, which is not only a danger to the cardiovascular system but also to the kidneys. High blood pressure is the second leading cause of kidney disease, as it forces the kidneys to filter at a higher rate, which over time places pressure on the kidneys, causing damage. To add to the insult, kidney damage also causes high blood pressure. So we certainly do not want to make matters worse by consuming foods that increase blood pressure further.

Obviously, this means not adding salt to meals and also avoiding fast foods and take-away, which usually contains a lot of salt for flavoring. But what many people are unaware of is that there are many foods that contain hidden sources of sodium. These include processed meats, frozen and canned foods, sports drinks and flavored and processed snacks.

Potassium is another mineral that is found in many foods, most of which are usually considered healthy. Potassium is an essential mineral that is required for nerve function, cardiac function and fluid balance, but when the levels in the blood are not correctly balanced this presents a danger in regard to these functions.

In the case of kidney damage, potassium levels can build up in the blood and can cause an imbalance of fluids and result in cardiovascular problems. For this reason, the renal diet requires that potassium be limited. The extent of this will depend upon blood test results. The foods highest in potassium include; tomato, potato, banana, nuts, seeds, pumpkin and chocolate. In cases of excessively high potassium levels, it may be necessary to perform a process to remove the potassium from vegetables, as it is not possible to avoid potassium completely.

Additionally, there's Phosphorus that needs to be limited in the renal diet. Phosphates are found in high levels in several foods including; dairy foods, meat, wheat, peanuts, legumes, chocolate, coconut, eggs, and beer. Many of these products should be avoided in a healthy renal diet for other reasons however it is important to be aware of phosphate levels in otherwise healthy foods such as eggs and legumes if phosphorus levels are high in the blood.

Phosphorus is an essential mineral and one of its most important functions is the formation of bones and teeth, as it is involved in the regulation of calcium. However, in the case of kidney damage, phosphorus builds up in the blood and can lead to osteoporosis as too much blocks absorption of calcium. High levels of phosphorus can also contribute to high blood pressure, which as we have seen is an extreme danger to the kidneys.

Other Concepts Involved In Renal Diet

One other concept of the best renal diet is following a predominantly alkaline diet. One of the functions of the kidneys is to balance the pH level of the blood and this does not occur effectively in kidney disease. So to take some of the pressure off the kidneys, removing acidic foods from the diet is a huge help, and will give the kidneys a chance to heal.

Meanwhile, acidity can contribute to a myriad of health issues throughout the body, many of which are associated with kidney problems. The wide list includes; kidney stones, urinary problems, high blood pressure, and poor immunity.

Now, following the alkaline diet is unfortunately not as simple as avoiding foods that taste acidic. It is the residue that is left once a food has been metabolized within the body that dictates whether or not that food is acidic. A good example of this is lemon. It tastes acidic but it actually produces an alkalizing effect once it is digested.

Generally speaking, most foods that are considered unhealthy are acidic so should be avoided regardless as part of the renal diet.

This includes meat, sugary treats, wheat, alcohol, and most dairy products. However, there are some acidic foods that are a healthy component of the renal diet, such as olive oil, fish, soymilk, and nuts.

But the good news is that this system is not too complicated. Initially, in the renal diet, you need to consume 80% alkaline and 20% acidic foods, so you can choose some of the healthy acidic options as part of your daily diet. It is possible to test your urinary pH daily, and once it has shown consistent improvement you can change to a maintenance diet of 60% alkaline and 40% acidic foods.

Most alkaline foods are considered healthy as part of the renal diet and include fruit and vegetables, brown rice, green juices, most herbal teas, tofu, and sprouts.

As you can see the best renal diet can vary depending upon your specific health problems and level of kidney damage, but there are some specific rules that it helps to be aware of. The appropriate renal diet is absolutely essential to both heal your kidneys and protect them from future damage. If you want to go even further to heal your kidneys there are many herbs and nutrients that have shown to improve kidney health.

The Do's and Don'ts of a Kidney Diet

If you are suffering from a renal problem such as kidney stones, then you may be interested to know that a kidney diet plays a significant part in mitigating adverse symptoms and helping the kidney recover quickly from the problem. While some foods may be very nutritious and good for the body, they may pose serious problems to the kidneys in the long run. Therefore, it is welladvised to eat meals in moderation and also evaluating the suitability of the diet to your condition.

A kidney diet should avoid calcium and phosphorous enriched foods

At best, dietary changes such as avoidance of calcium and phosphorous-rich foods will become necessary if certain kidney problems are at a critical stage. This applies mostly to individuals who are at risk of developing a renal disorder. Below are some of the do's and don'ts that you should consider when planning your kidney diet.

Don'ts of a kidney diet

+ Don't use food recipes in your diet for a renal disease which has substantial quantities of mineral salts especially oxalate salts from calcium, phosphorus, manganese. These mineral elements can cause faster kidney degeneration and severe impairment to kidney functioning.

✦ Don't eat excess portions of foods which have high concentrations of saturated fats such as fries, burgers, and red meat or any processed foods.

✦ Don't drink alcohol, energy drinks, or beverages with high sugar content-both may overwork the liver and worsen or cause degeneration of the kidney problem.

✦ Don't consume sugary substances such as snacks, desserts, or candies because they cause dehydration and overwork the kidney just like salts.

✦ Do not take all kinds of natural red meat in your kidney diet-beef, pork, bacon, or mutton and their alternatives fried, cured, or processed meats, instead look for lean white meat from poultry.

✦ Do not use any artificial sweeteners when preparing foods because they have no nutritional benefits

✦ Do not use margarine or mayonnaise but alternatives such as avocado fruit if you want to consume fat.

✦ Do not eat more helpings than necessary especially in regard to delicacies such as fries, ice creams, sodas, and other sweet foods an all kinds of processed or canned foods

+ Don't consume more carbohydrates than necessary in your kidney diet and this includes such carbs like pasta, white rice, biscuits, white sugar, white rice, and pasta.

Do's of a kidney diet

+ Do take enough fluids to keep the concentration of minerals such as calcium and sodium on the kidney low. These will to ensure proper kidney functioning, prevent dehydration which is the common cause of kidney stones in the renal tubes and detoxify the kidney as well.

+ Do adopt a balanced diet for a renal disease which comprises fresh vegetables, whole grains, and lean meat as well as water. Greens and fruits rich in vitamins improve cell metabolism and the functioning of organs.

+ Do take fiber or incorporate fiber-rich meals and whole grains in your renal diet which are low in carbs but promote general health and boost kidney functioning.

✦ Do eat moderately and develop healthy eating habits to ensure that your body gets the right supply of minerals and nutrients.

✦ Do eat vegetables and fruits as often as you can and incorporate them into your kidney diet plan to boost your immunity and cell metabolism

✦ Do use low-fat milk products such as milk powder if you have to use them instead of using milk with cream or fat.

✦ Do use monounsaturated fat or natural fat when cooking and lower the amount of fat that you consume per day in your meals.

✦ Do embrace active and vibrant life to reduce obesity or abnormal weight, boost the functioning of renal diet, and promote good body metabolism and kidney functioning. Exercise ensures blood circulation to kidney and boosts activities such as detoxification and filtering.

Undertaking a kidney diet is crucial to full recovery from your kidney problem. Not adhering to the guidelines could lead to the prolonging or worsening of the renal problem. Seek a doctor's advice before beginning any kidney diet program.

WHAT ARE THE BENEFITS OF A RENAL FAILURE DIET?

Kidney disease is a gradual loss of kidney function over a period of time, resulting in an accumulation of metabolic waste products in the body. The metabolic waste products and toxic substances are normally excreted by the kidneys. Based on the severity of the disease, kidney disease is classified into five stages. Stage 1 is the mildest and stage 5 is referred to as Renal Failure. In renal failure, there is a dangerous accumulation of water, waste and toxic substances in the body, that needs dialysis or renal transplantation to stay alive.

There are several dietary rules to follow; the renal failure diet helps to slow down the progress of renal failure. Normal kidneys remove toxins from the blood and regulate levels of sodium, potassium, and phosphorus. In renal failure, kidneys are unable to remove metabolic waste products and renal failure diet helps to regulate the amount of daily consumption of protein, fluids, sodium, potassium, and phosphorus.

PROTEIN - It is important to consume the appropriate amount of protein in renal failure, the protein intake is limited to 0.75 grams per kg body weight. Excessive intake of protein builds up metabolic waste products in the blood and there will be more work for the kidneys. In renal failure, more damage occurs to the kidneys if they are overworked. Less protein intake produces fewer waste products for kidneys to filter and kidney function can be preserved. On the other hand, protein consumption should not be too low which may cause muscle wasting. High-quality sources of protein include egg, lamb, poultry, fish, pork and beef.

FLUIDS - It is recommended to restrict fluid intake in renal failure because excessive fluid intake can cause fluid retention. Liquid foods such as soup, ice cream, contain water and certain vegetables and fruits contain more water which includes melons, lettuce, grapes, apples, and oranges. Consumption of such foods should be monitored because they add to fluid intake. The recommended quantity of fluid intake varies from patient to patient; a health care practitioner or a registered dietician can help to determine the appropriate amount of fluids required for a particular patient.

SODIUM - Sodium intake should be restricted in a patient with renal failure because excessive sodium intake can cause fluid retention leading to edema and hypertension. Rich sources of sodium include table salt, processed foods, and canned foods. It is advised to limit the consumption of packed chips, pickle, processed cheese, junk food, and smoked meat. Sodium intake should be less than 5 mg per serving.

POTASSIUM - The normal intake of potassium is 3.5 to 5.0 mEq/L and the consumption more than normal range should be avoided. Kidneys excrete about 90% of potassium consumed through the diet, excessive accumulation of potassium in the blood can cause life-threatening complications including cardiac arrhythmia. Patients are recommended to restrict potassium-rich foods such as yogurt, milk, citrus fruits, potatoes, tomatoes, dry fruits, bananas, beans nuts, and legumes.

PHOSPHORUS - The normal intake of phosphorus is 2.7 to 4.6 mg/dl, and excessive consumption should be avoided. Because increased blood phosphorus levels absorb calcium from the bone and cause bone diseases. Patients are advised to avoid phosphorous-rich foods such as cocoa, beer, dairy products, legumes, nuts, and meat.

Renal Diet - Controversial Diet That Kidney Patients Should Know About

A renal diet is a highly recommended diet for patients having renal problems. It is estimated that only 25% of the total number of nephrons are necessary to maintain healthy renal function. That means that the renal failure system is well protected from failure with a large backup system. However, it also means that by the time a patient has signs and symptoms of renal failure, extensive kidney damage have already occurred.

Dietary adjustment is dictated by many components including accumulation of nitrogenous waste products, impaired excretion of electrolytes, vitamin deficiencies and continued catabolism. Wasting syndrome is a major problem. The client with renal failure constantly loses body weight, muscle mass, and adipose tissue.

The purpose of this renal diet is to maintain a balance of electrolytes, minerals, and fluid in patients who are on dialysis.

This is important because dialysis alone cannot remove and filter all the wastes in the body. It needs a proper diet to aid the body in managing the accumulated wastes.

Dietary intake of electrolytes may be encouraged or restricted.

The regulation of sodium is a delicate matter. At times, the kidneys waste salt, and sodium intake must be encouraged to replace it. More frequently, however, the kidneys retain sodium.

Some believe that there should be a moderate restriction with careful monitoring of urinary sodium as a guideline. Another thing is the monitoring of fluid status which gives important information about sodium needs.

Renal failure and its therapies significantly affect the quality of the client and family members.

There can be numerous stressors and life changes. Much of the care required by clients receiving chronic peritoneal dialysis and hemodialysis and their significant others concerns the psychosocial aspects of dialysis

This is not like every diet out there. It is a carefully measured guide on how to approach the signs and symptoms of renal failure but still maintain an adequate amount of energy level to sustain your day to day activities. It also specifies the exact amount of dietary protein, electrolytes, minerals, and fluid that are allowable for each patient.

With the rampant spread of renal failure globally, it is understandable that a lot of renal diets have started to sprout out. There are also many scam sites out there who claim to have a "quick fix renal diet" so be careful. It is therefore important to do your research carefully and choose only websites that you deem trustworthy.

THE BENEFIT OF FOLLOWING THE CHRONIC RENAL FAILURE DIET TO SPEED RECOVERY FROM CHRONIC RENAL FAILURE

The popularity of chronic kidney failure diet has increased exponentially over time due to what research has shown to be against the backdrop of an increasing number of kidney disease failure patients, both diagnosed and undiagnosed. This special but easy to follow a simple diet of renal failure, when followed will drastically reduce the progression of the kidney disease and increase the rapidity rate of recovery.

The kidney disease condition called the chronic renal failure is a gradual but steady or consistent decline or loss of function of the kidney due to various arrays of insult on the kidney upon which the extent of damage depends.

Causes like pyonephrosis, nephrosclerosis, glomerulonephritis, obstructive kidney conditions due to blocking kidney stones and birth anomaly- congenital malformations, effects of some drugs especially when abused and over the use of pain killer have been implicated in the chronic renal failure disease.

For whichever cause, the result is always the same- retention of dangerous waste products/fluids of nitrogenous bases, causing electrolyte imbalance and death if unchecked.

As part of efforts to prevent the degeneration of the kidney disease to end-stage renal failure, the stage at which most

Americans with kidney conditions fear most, the chronic renal failure diet has become very imperative and indispensable. The diet depends on some factors like the patient nutritional status, medical method of treatment and condition. But whichever course and cause, the diet is simple to follow to achieve an optimum result.

The diet guide includes a cautious guideline on protein intake, fluid intake to balance fluid losses, sodium intake to balance sodium losses and some control over potassium-rich diets. At the same time, sufficient caloric intake and vitamin supplementation have to be ensured.

Protein Intake: should be of high biologic value including dairy products, eggs, and meats. Fluid allowance is between 500 to 600mL usually measured to be more than the previous day's urine output in a 24-hour check. Calories should be supplied from carbohydrate and fats to avoid muscle tissue wasting. Vitamin supplementation is also of critical importance as renal disease diets are always low in vitamin and hence supplementation is needed. In addition, the chronic renal failure patient who is on dialysis may likely lose water-soluble vitamins such as vitamin B complex and vitamin C from the blood during the dialysis treatment; hence the critical need for nontoxic vitamin supplementation.

In Chronic renal disease, the chronic renal failure diet is closely followed in line with medical advice and guide will certainly and positively help the patients' recovery rate to be enhanced without suffering drug complications or any adverse drug reactions or effects. This, together with proper medication will form the sure bet recovery synergy which neither medicines nor diet alone could achieve.

The Delicate Diet of a Renal Patient

Our kidneys, like the lungs, are paired organs that work equally to eliminate wastes in the body while removing excess water from the blood. Surprisingly, a human body could survive with one kidney alone and is able to live a normal life. No organ in the body could replace the function of the kidneys. There are certain instances that render the functions of both kidneys, making our bodies unable to process waste materials like urine. Kidney illnesses are characterized from mild to life-threatening problems. More often, people that suffer from kidney failures undergo a treatment called hemodialysis were the blood is being filtered via a machine, removing wastes materials that are poisonous to the body and getting rid of excess fluids in the blood. Some only use dialysis in a short period of time until their kidneys are able to function, while others with complete kidney failure, the procedure are a lifetime process. People that undergo dialysis are required to follow a strict diet. Sad to say there are a lot of restrictions regarding the diet of a renal patient.

Low sodium foods

A person who undergoes dialysis is not allowed to eat high sodium foods. Sodium attracts water like a magnet since the function of the kidneys of a renal patient is low to none, excess fluids inside the body is very deadly. Medical experts and doctors are very strict regarding the diet of a renal patient; they know that one wrong move could be fatal.

Low potassium foods

Potassium like sodium also attracts fluid in our body. Although they could cancel each other out excess quantities to both fluids would be unhealthy to renal patient.

Potassium-rich foods are very abundant to the market. We all know that fruits are very beneficial to our health, however, there are certain types of fruits that are not appropriate to a renal patient. Mangos, avocados, watermelons, and papaya are some of the potassium-rich fruits, while apple and pineapple are allowed in the diet of a renal patient. Carrots, celery, cucumber, red pepper, and green pepper are low potassium vegetables are included in the diet of the dialysis patient.

Restrict fluids

A renal patient is required to monitor his or her fluid intake, excess fluids could cause damage to remaining healthy organs in the body. Soups and Oatmeal should be taken in a minimal manner.

The diet of a renal patient is very fragile. We must familiarize ourselves of the allowed and not allowed foods, if not their conditions could worsen. The key to any diet is a balance; if we could attain that, our health would be secured.

KIDNEY FOODS DIET FOR HEMODIALYSIS

Damage to our kidneys can either be temporary or permanent, and either way, you most definitely do not want this to happen to your kidneys. Once our kidneys begin to fail, we experience a lot of symptoms that can be as subtle as a simple loss of appetite to even greater symptoms such as arrhythmias or even coma.

However, when you already have damaged kidneys and are undergoing hemodialysis there are still some kidney foods that you can take to better hasten the healing process of your kidneys. In choosing which food to include in your diet, you simply have to take note of certain nutrients that are essential for your speedy recovery.

Below is a list of nutrients that one should increase or decrease when undergoing hemodialysis.

Calcium and phosphorous usually work in adjunct to each other, and they actually do more than just keeping our teeth and bones strong. A change in one of these two nutrients will also affect the other. Usually, once your kidneys fail, phosphorous tends to build up in the blood. Having high levels of phosphorous in the blood is never a good thing because it can lead to a lot of problems such as brittle bones, or even heart damage. So it is a good idea to decrease your phosphorous intake while also taking calcium implements just to prevent certain complications.

Sodium is also one nutrient that should be limited in a renal diet. Limiting sodium intake can help to control blood pressure and fluid build up, which are common signs of kidney failure.

Sodium is commonly found in salt, so decrease intake of foods that are high in sodium such as processed foods, snack foods, and canned foods.

Usually when one is undergoing hemodialysis, one tends to lose a lot of proteins. As we all know, proteins are helpful in repairing tissues, fighting infection, and building muscles. So it is a good idea to increase your intake of food high in protein. Egg whites are a great source of proteins and they are much safer than meat.

These are only some of the nutrients that you should look for in kidney foods. Though it can be challenging to follow, keep in mind that well-nourished patients actually recover faster and at the same time have fewer chances of getting an infection.

Important Food Items to Cure Renal Diseases

It has been found after extensive medical research that free radicals are the source of any type of medical disorders including kidney problems. So foods containing antioxidants help to neutralize the effect of free radicals and thereby protect the body from harmful medical conditions. The renal diet incorporates kidney-friendly foods and is as follows:-

Red bell peppers

This food item is low in potassium content and high in vitamin A, vitamin C, vitamin B6, fiber and folic acid but high in flavor.

Most importantly they are the perfect items for a kidney diet.

This food item is rich in antioxidant lycopene that protects against certain forms of cancers. I used this item in salad as well as in omelets, and it tastes really good.

Cabbage

I am a very fond of the vegetable cabbage especially the green one. It has numerous nutritional contents in the form of phytochemicals and other chemical contents that help to break free radicals and thereby prevent the occurrence of any diseases. The contents present in this vegetable also help to prevent cardiovascular diseases as well as cancers from taking place. The presence of vitamin C, vitamin K, vitamin B6, folic acid, fiber, and low potassium and cost makes it an ideal kidney diet.

Cauliflower

It is yet another vegetable that is very common, affordable and an ideal kidney diet. The presence of vitamin C, fiber and compounds that neutralize toxic substances make this vegetable a healthy food item. I use this vegetable in large quantities, in salad, curry and truly speaking it tastes really good.

Garlic

Garlic has a number of health benefits. It contains chemicals like potassium, sodium, and phosphorus. Apart from being an excellent kidney diet, this food item lowers cholesterol, prevents plaque formation in the teeth as well as reduces inflammation. It imparts flavor to food items and therefore is widely used. Garlic is a part of my diet even today owing to its innumerable benefits.

Onions

These are the most common vegetables and are used in many delicious recipes. Onions contain elements like potassium, sodium, phosphorus, chromium, sulfur. It is sometimes eaten raw and at other times is used in salads, sandwiches. It is a good item to counter renal diseases.

Apples

Apples are extremely nutritious fruits, containing phosphorus, potassium. This food item reduces cholesterol, prevents the occurrence of any heart diseases as well as it prevents constipation. The fruit is ideal for a kidney diet.

Other Food Items That Forms a Part of the Renal Diet

The chronic kidney disease diet includes the above. Besides, there are other items that have taken as a part of the renal diet includes the following:-

+ Cranberries

+ Blueberries

+ Raspberries

+ Strawberries

+ Cherries

+ Red grapes ▪ Fish

+ Egg whites

+ Olive oil

Antony Jason Willfour

CHRONIC KIDNEY DISEASE (CHRONIC RENAL FAILURE/END STAGE RENAL

DISEASE) AND IT IS DIETARY MANAGEMENT

End-stage renal disease (ESRD) occurs when chronic kidney disease worsens to the point at which kidney function is less than 10% of normal. The kidneys fail to function at a level needed for day-to-day life. Kidneys main function is to remove wastes and excess of water from the body, which gets accumulated in renal failure leading to toxicity. The

148

treatment includes kidney transplant or dialysis with dietary management.

ESRD always follows a chronic kidney disease; the most common cause is diabetes and high blood pressure. Other causes are -

1. Diseases affecting arteries reaching or leaving the kidneys.
2. Congenital abnormalities of kidneys
3. Polycystic kidney disease
4. Too much abuse of pain medications or other drugs
5. Toxic chemicals
6. Autoimmune disorders like systemic lupus erythematosus (SLE), scleroderma
7. Injury
8. Glomerulonephritis
9. Kidney stones and secondary infections
10. Reflux nephropathy
11. Various other kidney diseases

Symptoms include -

1. General ill feeling and fatigue

2. Pruritis (itching) and dry skin

3. Weight loss without effort

4. Headache

5. Loss of appetite

6. Nausea and vomiting

7. Swelling

8. Bone pains

9. Bad breath

10. Abnormally dark skin

11. Changes in nails

12. Bleeding easily - bruises, nosebleed, blood in the stool

13. Impotence

14. Restless leg syndrome

15. Sleeplessness

16. Excessive thirst

17. Frequent hiccups

18. Amenorrhea

19. A drowsy and confused state

20. Cannot concentrate or think clearly 21. Numbness in different parts of the body

22. Cramps or twitching of muscles.

23. Abnormal health and lung sounds

24. Diminished or no urine production

ESRD leads to a buildup of waste products and fluid in the body, which affects most body systems and functions, including, blood pressure control, red blood cell production, electrolyte balance, vitamin D and calcium levels and thus bone health. Hence the patient on dialysis needs to undergo various tests often to manage the condition -

1. Sodium

2. Potassium

3. Phosphorus

4. Calcium

5. Magnesium

6. Albumin

7. Cholesterol

8. Electrolyte

9. Complete blood count (CBC)

10. Erythropoietin

11. Parathyroid hormone (PTH)

12. Bone density test

Treatment and Management

Management and treatment of ESRD include kidney transplant or dialysis and dietary management, it is essential for the patient to know and understand everything about the treatment especially about dialysis and its types.

Why dialysis - dialysis helps to remove and maintain waste products, fluid and the electrolyte balance in the body. A special diet is important as dialysis alone does not effectively remove all the waste products. And dietary management also helps minimize the amount of waste build-up and to maintain the fluid, electrolyte and mineral balance in the body between the dialysis.

One needs to do lots of changes in their diet -ESRD patients need high protein, low sodium, potassium and phosphorus diet, and restricted fluid intake. Let's consider each in little details -

Fluid

Urine output drops during kidney failure. Most dialysis patients urinate very little or not at all, and therefore fluid restriction between treatments is very important. Without urination, fluid will build up in the body and cause excess fluid in the heart, lungs, and ankles.

Your nutritionist will calculate the daily required amount of fluid on the basis of -

✦ The amount of urine output in 24 hours

✦ The amount of weight gain between the dialysis treatment

✦ Amount of fluid retention

✦ Levels of dietary sodium

✦ Whether you are suffering from congestive heart failure.

Tips -

✦ Avoid or minimize eating food with too much water like - soups, Jell-O, popsicles, ice creams, grapes, melons, palm fruit, coconut water, lettuce, tomatoes, and celery.

✦ Use smaller glasses.

✦ Take sips of water

✦ Minimize sodium intake. Avoid salty food

✦ Freeze juices in an ice tray and suck them to minimize thirst (do count these ice cubes in your daily fluid intake)

✦ Avoid getting too hot, going out in the sun.

Sodium balance -

As said above ESRD patient need to avoid high sodium diet. Hypertension in ESRD is mostly due to positive sodium balance and volume expansion (accumulation of too much fluid in the body).

ESRD patients on dialysis can effectively treat or control hypertension without antihypertensive drugs just by having a low sodium diet (2 g/day). Also, a low sodium diet will make you feel less thirsty and thus help avoid gulping extra fluids.

Tips -

+ Avoid - canned, processed food, processed smoked meat.

+ Avoid food with salt topping viz - chips, nuts, etc.

+ Read labels carefully - select one that reads - low sodium, no salt added, sodium free, unsalted.

+ Avoid foods that list salt near the beginning of the ingredient list.

+ Choose food which contains salt less than 100 mg per serving.

+ Remove the salt shaker from the table.

+ Cook food without salt instead use herbs for flavoring.

✦ Avoid preserved foods - ketchup, sauces, pickles, popadums

✦ Do not use salt substitutes, they contain potassium. And potassium is also restricted in kidney disease.

Potassium balance -

Normally a high potassium diet is recommended to control hypertension and thus minimize the risk of stroke and heart failure, but in case of ESRD, they cannot tolerate high potassium diet as they cannot excrete potassium from their body. High potassium levels in the blood will lead to life-threatening hyperkalemia induced arrhythmia.

Tips -

✦ Avoid fruits high in potassium - banana, musk melons, cantaloupes, kiwis, honeydew, prunes, nectarines, coconut water, tomatoes, avocado, oranges and orange juice, raisins, and dried fruits.

✦ Have fruits like - peaches, grapes, pears, cherries, apples, berries, pineapple, plums, tangerines, and watermelon.

✦ Avoid vegetables high in potassium - spinach, pumpkin, winter squash, sweet potato, potatoes, asparagus.

- ✦ Choose vegetables like - broccoli, cabbage, carrots, cauliflower, celery, cucumber, eggplant (aubergine/brinjal), green and waxed beans, lettuce, onion, peppers, watercress, zucchini, and yellow squash.

- ✦ Avoid legumes, milk and bran cereal.

- ✦ Limit intake of potassium up to 2 gm per day.

Iron -

Patients with ESRD will also need extra iron.

Tip -

- ✦ Consume food high in iron levels - lima and kidney beans, beetroot, green leafy vegetables (avoid spinach), finger millet, chicken, liver, pork.

- ✦ Eat iron-fortified cereals

- ✦ Take iron supplements as advised by your physician or dietician.

Calcium and phosphorus -

In ESRD phosphorous levels are high as it cannot be excreted from our body. Even in the early stages of renal disease, phosphorus levels can become too high. High phosphorus levels will lead to itching, vascular calcifications, secondary hyperparathyroidism, and low calcium levels. Thus the calcium deposited in the bones is used up leading to osteoporosis. Hence a phosphate restricted diet is recommended.

Tips -

+ Limit intake of dairy foods - milk, yogurt, and cheese.

+ Can consume dairy products like - margarine, butter, cream cheese, full-fat cream, brie cheese, and sherbet as they are low in phosphorus.

+ Consult your dietician and take calcium and vitamin D supplement, helps control calcium phosphate levels.

+ Avoid canned processed food.

If phosphorus levels are not managed with diet, your physician may prescribe you phosphorus binders.

Weight Management -

ESRD patient loses weight without any reason, thus their weight needs to be monitored and managed with a properly balanced diet. ESRD patients average calorie intake reduces to lower than 30-35 kcal/kg/day leading to malnutrition. To prevent malnutrition related morbidity and mortality, ESRD patients on dialysis need to undergo a periodic nutrition screening and tests, comparing initials body weight with usual and ideal body weight, dietary reviews, and food diary assessment. **Protein -**

You must be confused when I say ESRD patients need high protein, as most known fact is patients with renal diseases should limit their protein intake. True as when protein breaks down in our body urea is formed this cannot be excreted in urine and is toxic when it builds up in the bloodstream. This limited protein diet is until the patient is put on dialysis. As protein losses are higher in patients undergoing dialysis, they need to consume a high protein diet. Recommended dietary protein in hemodialysis patients is 1.2 g/kg body weight/day and 1.2-1.3 g/kg body weight /day for patients on peritoneal dialysis. If dietary protein - calorie intake is not adequate, patients should take dietary supplements under the guidance of a nutritionist, and if required they should be tube feed or parenteral nutrition should be provided.

Tips -

+ Eat high-quality protein - fish, pork, eggs, kidney beans, Bengal gram, and soy for every meal.

✦ Add egg white or egg white powder or protein powder to your diet.

Carbohydrates -

If you are overweight and have diabetes, then you have to limit your carbohydrate intake, however, if you are losing weight you need to take a high carbohydrate diet. As carbohydrates are a good source of energy. Your physician or dietician will recommend the number of carbs required in your diet.

Tips -

✦ Include - fruits, vegetables, bread, and grains, as they are high in fiber, minerals, vitamins and a good source of energy.

✦ If you are advised a high-calorie diet, consume - hard candies, sugar, honey, jelly, pies, cakes, cookies.

✦ Avoid desserts made from dairy, chocolate, nuts, and bananas.

Fats -

ESRD patients on dialysis are recommended to limit intake of saturated fats and cholesterol as they are at high risk of developing coronary artery disease. They mostly have high triglyceride levels, high LDL (low-density lipoproteins) and low HDL (high-density lipoproteins). Though you are recommended to eat a high-calorie diet, you need to avoid foods that raise your triglycerides and cholesterol levels

Tips -

✦ Include foods that are high in monounsaturated and polyunsaturated fats and little of saturated fats. Like - sesame seed oil, flaxseeds, olive oil, and cottonseed oil.

✦ Avoid canola oil, coconut oil, fats, poultry and chicken with skin.

Micronutrients -

ESRDS patients are recommended to have a low-fat diet and restricted fluid intake. Thus many patients need to take a vitamin supplement as fat-soluble (A, D, E, and K) vitamins and watersoluble vitamins cannot be absorbed adequately form the diet and water-soluble vitamins are also lost during dialysis treatment. Mostly these vitamins are given through vein during the dialysis treatment.

RENAL DIET - PREVENT KIDNEY FAILURE

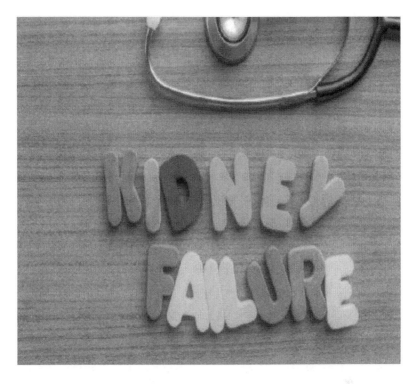

Chronic renal failure or chronic kidney diseases is the condition in which a person loses kidney function. Kidney has the functionality to eliminate toxins from the body but if the kidney fails to work properly, the body will start retaining fluid and the fluid quantity in the bloodstream will increase. In extreme case, the body swells and the functioning of lung and heart is affected.

Excess intake of water is flushed by the kidney but kidney failure or renal failure can result in a life-threatening condition in which the fluid is not eliminated from the body. To prevent such a condition one should follow strict dietary guidelines and follow a renal diet to control the buildup of wastages in the blood to reduce overload on the kidney. Some of the guidelines included in the renal diet are:

1. Sodium should be eliminated from the diet to prevent major damage and pressure on the kidney. One should reduce intake of beef, cured meat products, bacon, sausages, cheese, pickle, Chinese dishes and soy in the diet.

2. Canned food items such as vegetables, meat, shellfish, and processed meat should not be taken.

3. Low sodium food includes unprocessed meat and fish. Frozen or processed fruits and vegetables should not be taken.

4. The homemade soup should be taken. Preservatives used in cakes, biscuits or cheese have a high amount of sodium and it should not be taken. Most of the products which are made from baking powder contain sodium and to reduce intake of sodium, reduce intake of baked dishes.

5. Salt-free food items and butter should be included in the food.

6. People who suffer from kidney problem and take a good amount of fluid may suffer from swelling, breathlessness, high blood pressure and excess fluid can further deteriorate the condition of kidney. One should reduce intake of soda, coffee, tea, milk, coups, and ice creams.

In extreme case, the patient may suffer from renal failure and he/she may have to go on dialysis. Even on dialysis, it is advised to take a restricted diet to prevent further damage to the kidney. The following rules should be followed in case the patient goes on dialysis.

1. One should reduce intake of fluid and reduce the intake of a high salt diet. Salt products, potassium, certain electrolytes, phosphorus should not be taken in food and reduce the number of calorie intake to reduce weight.

2. Patients who are on dialysis may need more proteins as compared to a patient who is not on dialysis. On dialysis, the patient does not urinate or urinates very little.

3. The patient is asked to take a good amount of fruits and vegetables but most of the fruits or vegetables should have a low amount of potassium. Low potassium food items such as blackberries, plums, grapes, asparagus, beans, cucumber and summer squash should be included in the diet. The juices such as lemonade or apple juice can be taken but it should be taken in restricted quantities.

4. Phosphorus is found in food products such as nuts, dates, organ meat, dairy products, whole grains, coconuts, raisin and it should be avoided if a patient is on dialysis.

Chronic Kidney Disease Diet - Find Out What Doctors Don't Want You to Know About

Chronic kidney disease diet has become so popular nowadays simply because it has grown to be the trend in various races around the world. It is more prevalent in people nearing age 60 at about 40%, but kidney failure can show itself to people as young as 20.

The prevalence of chronic renal disease has increased by up to 25% from the previous decade. The increasing incidence of diabetes mellitus, hypertension high blood pressure, obesity, and an aging population have led to this increase in kidney disease.

Centers for Disease Control determined that almost 20 percent of all adults' above the age of 20 years old have chronic kidney disease. To put it into a harsher term, if you are on a bus with 9 other people, there are almost 1 of 5 chances that you have signs of having kidney disease. Now, this is one of those rare times when playing Russian roulette would seem to be a better alternative.

Scary isn't it?

CDC further indicates that over 400,000 patients are on dialysis or have received kidney transplants. This is a number that is expected to rise in the next decade as lifestyle and diet of today's John Doe is too much of what the body can effectively handle. To top it all off, about 67,000 people die each year because of kidney failure.

Here's how it gets controversial with the doctors:

The chronic kidney disease diet is usually done best before you have any renal diseases. It acts as a prophylactic measure in caring for your kidneys thereby making it healthy. However, like most people, we only come to realize the wrongness of our actions after we have experienced the consequences. As a nurse, many patients who later come to regret the abuse that they have done with their kidneys. They now experience chronic renal disease and must undergo weekly dialysis and await kidney transplantation.

Perhaps the best news that nephrology has to offer kidney patients is the fact that proven renal diets can be used as an adjunct to pre-dialysis and pre-transplantation treatment through adequately low protein diet, hypertension, anemia, and diabetes.

Its effectiveness has been supported by a lot of research studies both in the United States and the UK and has been proven to delay the progression of renal diseases by hundreds of patients who have used this method before you.

As the chronic kidney disease diet becomes more popular, it would be wise to evaluate your lifestyle and how you take care of your kidneys.

DO YOU HAVE CHRONIC RENAL DISEASE? KNOW THE SYMPTOMS

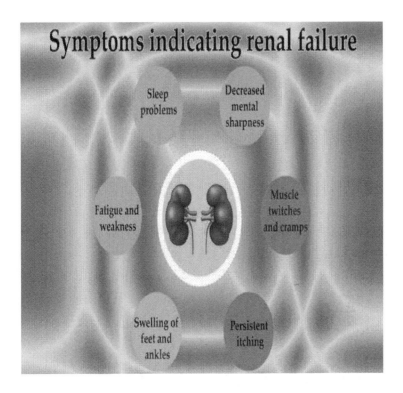

Your kidneys are probably not something you think about very often, but they are vitally important to how your body processes everything that you digest on a regular basis. Every time you eat a meal, drink beverages or alcohol, take vitamins, prescription medication or drugs, your kidneys are hard at work processing all of that, disposing of unneeded waste, filtering your blood and monitoring your body's natural acidity level (PH). It's the silent workhorse that is easy to ignore until something goes wrong.

Studies show that 1 in 9 American adults have some form of medical renal disease or kidney failure. Renal is the Latin word for kidney, so when you hear your doctor talking about renal problems, he or she is discussing the state of your kidneys. Renal (or kidney) disease has reached epic proportions in America, especially with the rise of obesity and diabetes. Both conditions are directly linked to chronic renal failure (CRF).

This is often called a silent disease because it's really hard to detect in its early stages. Most people only discover they have it during a later stage of the disease. Unfortunately, many don't get diagnosed until they are at the stage where they need dialysis or a kidney transplant. When caught earlier, it is treatable, so that's why it's important for you to know some of the symptoms that come with this condition.

In general, there are five stages of renal failure:

✦ Stages 1 and 2 - There will be mild kidney damage.

✦ Stage 3 - There is moderate kidney damage.

✦ Stage 4 - There is a severe decrease in kidney functions.

✦ Stage 5 - There is acute kidney damage and drastic life-saving measures are needed.

In the early stages, you will probably not notice much of anything. However, as the disease progresses, more symptoms will reveal themselves, such as frequent urination, or the opposite, urinating less than you normally do, bloating of hands, face, ankles and abdomen, headaches, itchy skin and feeling lethargic.

These symptoms will develop gradually as your kidneys slowly degenerate over a period of time. This is what makes it a chronic condition.

As long as you are not at the end stages of the disease, you can regain normal kidney function by making some strict dietary changes. There is a diet plan that addresses chronic renal failure and the toxins building up in your system. Your kidneys may fail for a variety of reasons, but this failure guarantees that they will be unable to process all the toxins that are accumulating in the bloodstream. Without this filtering, you will increasingly become ill. It is now known that people with chronic renal failure have abnormally high levels of phosphorous in their body. You will also have accumulated too much protein. Your health will continue to degenerate because of this build up.

Since you are getting most of your phosphorous and protein from the foods you eat, the number of foods that contain these elements will need to be greatly reduced. A good chronic renal disease diet plan will give you a list of foods that you can eat, and recommend that you do not eat others. You may have to consult with your physician or a dietitian before beginning such a diet, especially if you're already being treated for diabetes or heart disease.

Monitoring Your Protein Intake

As you already know the human body needs protein in order to function normally. Protein contains a lot of nutritional benefits and helps build muscle tissue and red blood cells. However, when the kidneys break down, they can no longer process protein as they normally do, so it starts building up in your bloodstream. In order to get your protein levels back down to normal, you'll have to eat a lot fewer meats and other foods that contain protein. In order to keep your energy levels up at all times, you can add a protein supplement to your everyday diet that won't conflict with your meals.

Foods with Low Phosphorous

Part of the kidney's job is to regulate the amount of phosphorous in your blood. When they can't do this normally, your phosphorous levels increase. These high levels of phosphorous decrease the amount of calcium in your blood. Calcium is necessary for healthy teeth and bones. When you lose calcium, your bone density decreases, which puts you at a greater risk for developing osteoporosis.

That's why the end-stage renal disease diet will show you which low phosphorous foods you should be eating to correct this problem. Some of the foods on the list of things you are allowed to eat are: cottage cheese, rice milk, cabbage, eggplant, white bread, crackers, pasta, beef, poultry, fish (except pollock, walleye salmon or sardines), potatoes, green peas, onions, cucumbers, bagels, white rice, broth-based soups, mayonnaise, salad dressing, butter, margarine, sherbet, ginger ale and hard candy.

Some of the foods you'll be giving up are: milk (including soy milk), hard cheese, ice cream, foods made from whole grains, soup containing milk, peas or beans, cornbread, biscuits, sweet potatoes, pumpkin, broccoli, mushrooms, spinach, asparagus, organ meats like liver, cream (all varieties), sesame butter, sour cream, soft drinks (except root beer and lemon-lime soda) and chocolate.

As you can see, this is an eating plan that excludes many foods that you probably enjoy eating. But, when it comes to your kidneys, they are so important to the quality of your life, that you should be willing to do anything to get them back to a normal state. The alternative is to ignore the problem until it becomes too late to do anything but hook you up to a dialysis machine.

While this would save your life, it's not an ideal situation. There are many end-stage renal failure patients who must spend every two to three days in the hospital getting a dialysis treatment. Too many of them are on a long waiting list to receive a kidney transplant.

By making some simple dietary changes, you (or a loved one you know with this disease), can avoid that fate and turn things around while there is still time. If you feel that you have even one of the above symptoms, make an appointment to see your doctor for a full kidney evaluation. The sooner you find out that you have chronic renal disease, the sooner you can take action to solve the problem.

Acute Renal Failure - Symptoms, And Treatment

Acute renal failure (ARF) is a very serious, but treatable condition, and is a result of the loss of kidney function.

There are various symptoms and treatments for acute renal failure or otherwise known as Acute Kidney Failure, or Acute Kidney Injury.

So What is Acute Renal Failure?

Acute kidney failure, as stated before, is the sudden loss of kidney function. As you may well be aware, your kidneys are responsible for removing waste products from the body and help to balance other minerals in your body and bloodstream. They are an essential part of the body, as the body can not work at all without them. With acute kidney failure, if your kidneys stop working, your body will soon build up with a large number of waste products, toxins, and other fluids and can, as a result, turn fatal.

How is Acute Renal Failure Caused?

There are various causes of acute renal failure. Some of which related to other causes in the body, which can affect the kidneys, while others are directly related.

Blockage of urine flow.

This can cause kidney failure by blocking the excretion of waste in the kidneys. It can be caused by a tumor, swollen prostate, urinary tract blockage or infection, an injury, or very commonly - kidney stones.

Loss of blood flow to the kidneys.

Any type of bodily injury, but more specifically, localized injuries to the kidneys can cause sudden blood flow loss, which can result in serious damage to the kidneys. This can also be the result of an infection, commonly known as sepsis. Extended dehydration can also cause serious damage. Certain medications can cause acute kidney failure.

There are some medications, which can have some very large side effects on the kidneys. This is not a related medication, but usually from people suffering other extended illnesses. Many of these types of medications can be found in some antibiotics, blood pressure medications, certain dyes used in CT scans, and more commonly some pain killers. All of these can have a poisoning effect on the kidneys and must not be taken for extended periods of time. If you suffer from any of these conditions, it is important to try to find other means of coping, including finding ways to fix the first cause of the problem.

Who is at risk of Acute Kidney Failure?

Some people may be more at risk of acute kidney failure. For those suffering chronic conditions such as heart conditions, obesity, liver disease, high blood pressure, and other organ conditions, they will have more chance of suffering from acute renal failure.

Again, as mentioned earlier, it is essential to look at ways to reduce stress on the kidneys if suffering the above condition to help avoid any chances of acute renal failure or kidney disease.

What are the common symptoms of Acute Renal Failure?

Prior to any form of kidney disease being clear, symptoms can be seen to be very mild, and may even remain unnoticed by some until it is too late. It is important that if you have any of these common symptoms, to act immediately. Common symptoms of acute renal failure may include fluid retention (swelling in the body - usually the feet and hands), loss of appetite, urinating problems, some vomiting and nausea, dizziness, pain in the lower back and general feelings of restlessness. For people who are already suffering other long-term medical conditions, these symptoms may go unnoticed and may be thought to be related to the current illness. It is important to remember that the slightest sign of acute renal failure symptoms, steps must be taken to help treat the condition.

How is tell if you have Acute Kidney Failure

Acute kidney failure is determined by simple medical tests. On consultation of your symptoms with your doctor, urine and blood samples must be taken. These can help show the toxicity of your blood and urine and can help decide if you are now at risk of acute renal failure. Other tests such as monitoring your fluid intake and loss are very important, to help indicate if there is any fluid retention being caused.

How to treat Acute Kidney Failure

Acute renal failure has some forms of treatment which require hospital stays and ongoing treatments. This is all dependent on the severity of the acute renal failure and the symptoms or causes of renal problems. These treatments can range from dialysis, medications, and surgery. Depending on how far along the renal failure is will depend upon which treatment is selected. Many doctors are now discovering, however, that acute renal failure is primarily caused due to poor nutrition and lifestyle factors, as with almost all medical conditions. Some of our preferred western foods contain preservatives and chemicals that are not able to be processed by our body.

Along with this, it usually contain large amounts of sodium, and potassium, which are not at all good for anyone battling with kidney disease. The kidney diet was created based on eastern diets (who now have very rare cases of genetic-related renal failure) and has proven to help treat and even reverse the onset of acute kidney failure.

WHAT IS RENAL DIALYSIS?

Blood in tubing flows through dialysis fluid

Blood pump

Vein

Artery

Shunt

Used dialysis fluid

Air detector

Dialysis machine

Fresh dialysis fluid

Compressed air

Renal dialysis, or kidney dialysis, is the physical filtering procedure used to artificially remove waste products and excess water from the bloodstream.

The kidneys are the filtering organs that generally perform this task for us. They control the salt, electrolyte and fluid balance in the bloodstream necessary for all the systems in the body to function properly.

If the kidneys become damaged or diseased and their filtering ability compromised, toxins and water accumulate in the bloodstream and will eventually poison the person if nothing is done to help them.

Renal dialysis is used as a bridging procedure until either the kidney functions are restored, or the patient gets a kidney transplant.

In the case of renal disease, the kidney's filtering mechanism becomes damaged, inefficient and inaccurate. Some molecules such as blood cells and some proteins are passed into the urine and excreted, while dangerous salts and water are often retained.

Renal dialysis does not work as efficiently as a healthy kidney, but it does remove the most dangerous salts and the excess water accumulated in the body.

Dialysis does not cure kidney disease, it merely performs the most basic functions of the kidney necessary for the body to continue living normally. Dialysis has to be repeated at frequent intervals.

There are two basic types of renal dialysis, hemodialysis, and peritoneal dialysis. The principle behind the dialysis is that salts and water can pass through a semi-permeable membrane from one container to another. When the specific salt solutions are mixed in the correct concentration, they can "draw" other salts and water to themselves.

The dialysis fluid used is scientifically formulated to do just this. In hemodialysis, blood from the patient is taken via a tube in their arm, into a machine. In the machine, the blood flows on one side of the membrane and the dialysis fluid is pumped on the opposite side and in the opposite direction. The blood is thus cleansed and flows back into the patient.

The process takes up to 3 to 5 hours and is necessary at least 2 to 3 times a week. Most people needing hemodialysis have to attend a day center where it is performed. The whole procedure is very disruptive to the lifestyle of dialysis patients.

Peritoneal dialysis is usually performed at home. It is far less disruptive to lifestyle but needs to be performed at least daily or preferably twice a day. A special connection is inserted into the patient's peritoneum (abdominal cavity). The patient himself then attaches the dialysis mixture and allows it to flow in.

The peritoneum or mucus lining of the abdominal cavity is full of blood vessels, it acts as the membrane between the blood vessels and the dialysis fluid. The fluid is left in the peritoneum for a few hours, allowing it to do its work, then it is drained out and discarded. Peritoneal dialysis is not as efficient as hemodialysis, but, because it is done more frequently, the results are on a par.

Renal dialysis is a life-saving procedure to filter toxins and excess fluids out of the bloodstreams of patients suffering from damaged and diseased kidneys. Dialysis helps restore the electrolyte and water balances the body requires to function efficiently, so patients with severe renal damage can continue to live relatively normal lives when their kidneys fail.

Renal Dialysis Diet - What You Really Need to Know About Renal dialysis diet is recommended to patients who are undergoing dialysis. The purpose of this diet is to maintain a balance of electrolytes, minerals, and fluid in patients who are on dialysis.

The special diet is important because dialysis alone does not effectively remove ALL waste products. These waste products can also build up between dialysis treatments.

On the other side of the coin, renal dialysis is an artificial process by which waste products and excess fluid are removed from the body by diffusion from one fluid compartment to another across a semipermeable membrane.

Active or mechanical dialysis cycles blood through a machine (dialyzer) or cycles dialyzing fluid into and out of the client's abdominal cavity (peritoneum) through a semipermeable membrane to remove impurities and toxins and to maintain fluid, electrolyte and an acid-base balance. Passive dialysis uses the client's peritoneal membrane as the filter.

Acute renal failure may require dialysis until the client's kidney function improves and starts filtering the client's blood independently. ESRD is defined as irreversible, chronic renal failure requiring regular dialysis or a kidney transplant to sustain life.

There are two types of dialysis procedures in common clinical usage: hemodialysis and peritoneal dialysis. Both of them requires renal dialysis diet as a supplementary course of action.

During the hemodialysis process, blood passes through an artificial kidney machine and the waste products diffuse across a synthetic membrane into a bath solution known as dialysate after which the cleansed blood is returned to the client's body.

Hemodialysis is accomplished usually in three- to four-hour sessions, three times a week.

Occasionally, medical complications occur where a client retains more fluid than is healthy following regular dialysis treatment.

Ultrafiltration is a process of removing excess fluid from the blood through a dialysis membrane by exerting pressure. This procedure is part of hemodialysis treatment and is included in the composite rate for the hemodialysis treatment. Ultrafiltration is not a substitute for dialysis.

During the peritoneal dialysis process, waste products pass from the client's body through the peritoneal membrane into the peritoneal (abdominal) cavity where the dialysate is introduced and removed periodically.

Renal dialysis diet is used as an adjunct to patients undergoing dialysis. This special diet will also help you maintain proper fluid and electrolyte levels in between dialysis treatments.

Coupled with dialysis, it will effectively help you feel as good as possible and lessen complications from the build-up of toxins from having renal disease.

RENAL STONES

Some larger stones may block the flow of urine.

Individuals with renal stones present with flank pain and hematuria with or without having a fever. Based on the level of the rock and also the patient's underlying anatomy (e.g., if there is only an individual working kidney or significant preexisting renal illness), the presentation might be complicated by obstruction with decreased or absent urine production.

Even though a range of disorders may outcome in the improvement of renal stones, a minimum of 75% of renal stones contains calcium.

Most instances of calcium stones are due to idiopathic hypercalciuria, with hyperuricosuria and hyperparathyroidism as other major causes. Uric acid stones are typically caused by hyperuricosuria, especially in individuals with a history of gout or excessive purine consumption (eg, a diet plan higher in organ meat products).

Defective amino acid transport, as occurs in cystinuria, can outcome in stone creation. Lastly, struvite stones, made up of magnesium, ammonium, and phosphate salts, are the outcome of chronic or recurrent urinary tract infection by urease-producing organisms (usually Proteus). Renal stones outcome from alterations in the solubility of various substances in the urine, such that there are nucleation and precipitation of salts. A number of factors can tip the balance in favor of rock creation.

Dehydration favors rock formation, along with high fluid intake to maintain a daily urine volume of a couple of L or a lot more seems to be defensive. The precise mechanism of this protection is unknown. Hypotheses include dilution of unfamiliar substances that predispose to stone formation and decreasing the transit time of Ca2+ through the nephron, minimizing the likelihood of precipitation.

A high-protein diet plan predisposes to a rock formation in susceptible people. A dietary protein load causes transient metabolic acidosis and an elevated GFR. Even though serum Ca2+ is not detectably elevated, there is most likely a transient improve in calcium resorption from bone, an improve in glomerular calcium filtration, and inhibition of distal tubular calcium resorption. This effect appears to be greater in known stone-formers than in wholesome controls.

A high-Na+ diet plan predisposes to Ca2+ excretion and calcium oxalate rock formation, whereas a reduced dietary Na+ intake has the opposite effect. Furthermore, urinary Na+ excretion raises the saturation of monosodium urate, which can act as a nidus for Ca2+ crystallization. Despite the truth that most stones are calcium oxalate stones, oxalate concentration in the diet is generally as well low to assistance a recommendation to avoid oxalate to avoid stone creation.

Similarly, calcium restriction, formerly a main dietary recommendation to calcium rock formers, is beneficial only towards the subset of individuals whose hypercalciuria is diet plan dependent. In others, decreased nutritional calcium might actually improve oxalate absorption and predispose to rock creation.

A number of elements are defensive against rock creation.

In order of decreasing importance, fluids, citrate, magnesium, and nutritional fiber appear to use a defensive impact. Citrate might prevent rock formation by chelating calcium in solution and forming extremely soluble complexes in comparison with calcium oxalate and calcium phosphate.

Even though pharmacologic supplementation from the diet with potassium citrate has been shown to improve urinary citrate and pH and decrease the incidence of recurrent rock formation, the benefits of the naturally high-citrate diet plan have not been investigated. Nevertheless, some studies suggest that vegetarians use a lower incidence of stone formation.

Presumably, they avoid the stone-forming impact of high protein and Na+ within the diet plan, combined using the defensive effects of fiber along with other factors. Rock formation per se within the renal pelvis is painless until a fragment breaks off and travels down the ureter, precipitating ureteral colic. Hematuria and renal harm can occur in the absence of pain.

The discomfort associated with renal stones is due to distention from the ureter, renal pelvis, or renal capsule. The severity of discomfort is related to the degree of distention that happens and thus is extremely severe in acute obstruction. Anuria and azotemia are suggestive of bilateral obstruction or unilateral obstruction of an individual working kidney.

The pain, hematuria, as well as ureteral obstruction caused by a renal stone, are typically selflimited. For smaller stones, passage usually demands only fluids, bed rest, and analgesia. The major complications are (1) hydronephrosis and permanent renal harm as a result of total obstruction of the ureter, with resulting backup of urine and buildup of pressure; (a couple of) infection or abscess creation behind a partially or completely obstructing stone, which could rapidly destroy the involved kidney; (three) renal harm subsequent to repeated kidney stones; and (4) hypertension resulting from elevated renin production by the obstructed kidney.

WHAT IS A DIABETIC RENAL DIET?

For diabetics who also suffer from kidney disease, there is a food plan known as the diabetic renal diet. More than half of the sufferers of chronic kidney disease are people who are also diabetics, indicating the necessity for diabetics to follow the diabetic renal diet. In a number of cases, this diet is prepared for people who are already suffering from renal failure and are at different stages of the disease. There are also cases in which the diet is created for those diabetics hoping to avoid getting the renal disease. Sufferers of diabetes and kidney problems usually have trouble eating the right food.

The main purpose of a diabetic meal plan is to have the blood glucose levels consistently within the safe range. This can be done just by having meals regularly every day, not missing any of the meals, and eating carbohydrate foods which are low glycemic.

Consuming the same quantity of such carbohydrates at every meal can assist the body to have a constant level of blood glucose without it getting too high nor too low, and becoming uncontrollable. Low glycemic foods can be whole grain bread, sweet potatoes, and brown rice. However, if it is a renal diet for diabetics, whole grain bread and sweet potatoes ought not to be used because they are rich in potassium.

For people with kidney problems, they should eat less of those foods rich in phosphorus, potassium, and sodium. Blood glucose lowering diet for the diabetics can also be a diet suitable for renal problems. Since sodium is common in many foods, patients need to look at labels and choose foods which are low in sodium.

Dietitians for kidney problems advice against the consumption of diet sodas of the dark-colored variety and coffee since such drinks contain too much sodium for diabetics with renal problems to take regularly.

On a diabetic, renal meal plan, unsweetened teas, water, and clear diet sodas are allowed. When it comes to vegetables, broccoli, cauliflower, beets, eggplant, and cabbage are usually recommended due to their rich vitamin content and low carbohydrate and potassium content. Meats which are rich in sodium, such as organ meats, sausage and bacon ought not to be taken.

Since canned vegetables contain lots of sodium, it is really necessary to choose raw vegetable and avoid canned vegetables in a diabetic renal diet. Furthermore, raw vegetables are more nutritious with a greater amount of vitamins. It is recommended that diabetics with renal problems learn from certified nutritionists the foods they ought to eat and those they should avoid. Such a nutritionist can also provide knowledge on portion sizes which is important as it helps in blood glucose control.

Diabetic Renal Diet

Formulating the basics of a diabetic renal diet is a very important issue as diabetes is the single biggest cause of renal failure. Many people suffering from kidney problems are also diabetics.

Combining a renal diet with a diabetic diet has a number of challenges. Looking for an acceptable diet for both kidney failure and diabetes can appear to be very limiting to the patient at first.

The main objective for a diabetic diet is to maintain healthy sugar levels in the blood at all times. **There are basically two ways of achieving this:**

+ By only eating carbohydrates with a low GI (glycemic index) because they are broken down and absorbed more slowly resulting in a steady release of sugar into the bloodstream over a longer period of time. Low GI foods include whole grains, unrefined foods, most fruits and vegetables, legumes, sweet potatoes, and nuts. Highly refined and concentrated carbohydrates, like white bread, confectionaries, sugars, and drinks with added sugar should be avoided. They cause blood sugar "spikes", because they are very rapidly absorbed, and tend to burn out just as quickly.

✦ Eating small frequent meals (about 6 times a day is generally accepted). It is important to remember that it is not only what is eaten, but when it is eaten that keeps the blood sugar levels more constant. Don't go long periods without eating, and don't eat huge meals or skip meals.

✦ The renal diet, on the other hand, tries to limit stress on the kidneys by reducing waste products in the bloodstream:

✦ By limiting daily protein intake. Excess proteins eaten have to be broken down into carbohydrates and nitrites. The nitrites in the form of urea are eliminated in the urine. This causes unnecessary work for already damaged kidneys.

✦ Limiting table salt to avoid water retention. Salt replacements should not be used as they contain potassium.

The possible need to reduce other salts such as potassium and phosphates. These are monitored by frequent blood tests and only need to be limited to the advice of your doctor. Foods with high potassium content include apricots avocado, banana, cantaloupe, kiwi, citrus fruits, papaya, pears, peaches, prunes, and watermelon. Some foods with high phosphorus content are legumes, dairy, dried legumes, shellfish, organ meats.

Diabetic Renal Diet:

- Limit protein intake to approximately 8 oz, or two moderate servings, a day • Eat only low GI carbohydrates • Limit salt, to cooking only.
- Limit foods with high phosphorus and potassium contents, follow your Doctor's advice on this at all times.
- Eat small frequent meals. When you wake up in the morning, eat your first meal. Eat at 23 hourly intervals throughout the day, taking your last meal at bed-time.

Tips:

- Planning menus for a week at a time will help you vary your food more.
- Plan your daily food intake so it is spread throughout the day

+ When dishing up food for your main meal, fill half the plate with vegetables or salads, then the other half equally with carbohydrates and protein.

+ Instead of salt, add flavor by using fresh herbs, non-salt spices, onions, garlic, a little lemon juice or flavored oils.

+ For smaller meals eat whole grain cereal, crackers or bread, fruit, a glass of skim milk, nuts, yogurt, a little cottage cheese and plenty of salads.

A diabetic renal diet can be a very powerful aid in controlling both renal failure and diabetes. It is well worthwhile planning your eating and sticking to your diet. You will feel better and be healthier for it.

A healthy lifestyle that includes a balanced diet and exercise is recommended for everyone. For the diabetic these are essential.

The demands on the diet are extensive and comprehensive for the diabetic person. A renal diabetic diet is recommended for most patients, but there is no one set diet for everyone. The amounts and kinds of foods consumed will vary widely from person to person. The key is to adapt to the renal diabetic diet to the patient's individual need.

Diabetes cannot be cured as of today, but it can be controlled through a well-managed diet.

Maintaining a healthy weight is vital for diabetics. A renal diabetic diet can help get the patient to the right weight and help maintain it. Obesity or weight gain will cause diabetic symptoms to worsen and cause other health problems with kidneys and other organs. Not only obesity but a constantly fluctuating weight can also cause problems for the diabetic. Being able to maintain the right amount of insulin in the body becomes difficult when their weight keeps changing. A consistent renal diabetic diet helps level out these fluctuations and maintains the right amount of insulin.

Any diabetic can eat most foods, but depending on the severity and type of diabetes they have, it may be necessary to limit the amounts of certain foods. This list may include sugars, carbohydrates and fats, especially trans-fats. Alcohol should be avoided, but may be consumed in small amounts and only on occasion. In general, the amount of food consumed and the timing of meals needs to be closely monitored. This is the key benefit of the renal diabetic diet.

If you have been diagnosed with diabetes, you need to work with a physician and nutritionist to develop a customized diet as soon as possible to get your to condition under control. Diabetes is an on-going condition that cannot be cured. You will not outgrow it.

Even Type I, juvenile diabetes, will not be outgrown. Following a strict diet is the only way to manage this condition. Type II diabetes, adult onset, many times can be managed by only changing your diet. Following a great renal diet may be all you need to do.

Sometimes you will need to follow the diet and take oral medication. Sometimes you will need a renal diabetic diet and daily insulin injections. But no matter what your doctor recommends, be sure to follow the prescribed renal diabetic diet for your continued good health.

Diabetes is a medical condition whereby the human body produces an insufficient amount of insulin. Insulin is a natural hormone produced in the body. It is responsible for converting sugar, starch, and other food material into energy. Renal diabetes is a type of diabetes, which occurs due to a low-sugar threshold in the kidneys. Diabetic patients have to take special care about their food habits. Doctors typically prescribe a special renal diabetic diet for a diabetic patient.

A renal diabetic dietary chart specifies the type and amount of food that a patient should consume every day. A person suffering from renal diabetes should eat meals that contain the right amount of nutrients. The diets should have sufficient vegetables and leguminous fruits. Doctors also recommend a diet that has vegetables with low carbohydrate levels, such as celery and cucumbers. Foods rich in amino acids such as soybeans, red beans, eggs, and lean meat are also beneficial. Food that reduces the level of sugar in the bloodstream is very effective in the prevention and treatment of diabetes.

It is also critical for a diabetes patient to maintain proper body weight, as it helps in controlling blood fats (cholesterol) and lowering the blood pressure. A renal diabetic diet is designed to ensure that a diabetic does not gain weight.

People suffering from renal diabetes should avoid or eat very small quantities of any food that contains a high amount of cholesterol. They should also try to reduce their intake of fish, egg yolks and fatty meats. The use of fat or oil in cooking should be restricted. They should only consume food products with low levels of potassium. Artichokes, beans, Brussels sprouts, lentils, lima beans pumpkin, squash, spinach, succotash, and tomatoes are a few of the vegetables that are in a renal diabetic diet.

Renal diabetics can easily control their sugar level and lead normal lives by sticking to a renal diabetic diet.

DIABETIC RENAL DIET - HOW TO EFFECTIVELY MANAGE RENAL DISEASE

AND DIABETES

Being that one of the most common extrarenal diseases affecting the kidney is diabetes mellitus, the diabetic renal diet has become a topic of interest nowadays.

Diabetic nephropathy, a progressive process, commonly leads to renal failure. About 30% of clients with end-stage renal disease have diabetes mellitus.

Researchers estimate that 25% to 50% of clients with insulin- dependent diabetes mellitus or type 1 diabetes have to end-stage renal disease within 10 to 20 years of beginning insulin therapy.

Renal disease can also occur in the non-insulin dependent diabetic client. The incidence of proteinuria (protein in urine) is about 25% after the 20 years of diabetes.

This diabetic renal diet is a nutritional therapy to emphasize the need for a team approach to enhance the ability of each patient with diabetes to achieve good metabolic control. In this way, by controlling diabetes mellitus, we can manage the progressive worsening condition to our kidneys thereby preventing end-stage renal disease.

The kidney metabolizes 30% to 40% of insulin, and as renal function decline, the degradation of insulin also decreases, resulting in a lower insulin requirement. Renal failure may be initially identified when the client is evaluated for recurrent insulin reactions.

Researchers hope that exacerbation of renal disease can be slowed by the following:

+ Carefully controlling hypertension.

- Adjusting insulin therapy and carefully monitoring blood glucose to maintain normal sugar level.

- Restricting dietary protein.

Regardless of diabetic control, however, renal failure inevitably develops within 5 to 10 years after the appearance of significant proteinuria.

These are some recommended dietary modification for patients with diabetes mellitus:

Total calories- sufficient to maintain/achieve reasonable weight in adults, or meet increased needs of children, adolescents, pregnant and lactating women and individuals recovering from catabolic illness.

- Caloric distribution of 50- 70% of carbohydrates, 20- 30% of proteins and 20- 30% of fat.

- Cholesterol limit to 300 mg/day or less.

- Carbohydrates and sweetness

- Sodium limit to about 300mg/day, less for people with hypertension if renal complications.

- Alcohol- moderate amounts may be allowed, contingent on good metabolic control.

✦ Vitamin and mineral supplement- not necessary but may be given to individuals on reduced calorie diets (1200kcal/day or less)

There is no one diabetic diet that will suit the individual and the special need of a person with diabetes. The diet for an individual with diabetes can only be defined as a "dietary prescription based on nutrition assessment and treatment goals".

However, the diabetic renal diet can serve as a guideline on how to manage and control diabetes mellitus thus prolonging renal disease.

Renal Failure And Renal Diet - Save Yourself!

When it comes to your health and well being, it's a good idea to see your doctor as often as possible to make sure you don't run into preventable problems that you needn't catch. The kidney is your body's toxin filter (as is the liver), cleaning the blood of foreign substances and toxins that are released from things like preservatives in the food and other toxins.

When you eat irresponsibly and fill your body with toxins, either from food, drinks (alcohol for example) or even from the air you breathe (free radicals are in the sun and transfer through your skin, through dirty air, and many foods contain them). Your body also tends to convert many things that seem benign until your body's organs convert them into things like formaldehyde due to a chemical reaction and morphing phase.

One example of this is most of those diet sugars used in diet sodas for example, Aspartame turns into Formaldehyde in the body. These toxins have to be removed or they can lead to disease, renal (kidney) failure, cancer, and various other painful problems.

What is renal or kidney failure? This is when your kidneys are not capable of ridding the body of the toxins and wastes in your blood from the foods you eat and the things you drink. This is also called "chronic kidney disease" or "chronic renal failure".

This is not a condition that happens overnight- it is a progressive problem and in that it can be both discovered early and treated, diet changed, and resolving what is causing the problem is possible. It's possible to have a partial renal failure but usually, it takes a lot of time (or really bad diet for a short time) to reach total renal failure. You don't want to reach total renal failure because this will require regular dialysis treatments to save your life.

Dialysis treatments specifically clean the blood of waste and toxins in the blood using a machine because your body can no longer do the job. Without treatments, you could die a very painful death. Renal failure can be the result of long term diabetes, high blood pressure, irresponsible diet, and can stem out of other health concerns.

A renal diet is about moderating the intake of protein and phosphorus in your diet. Limiting your sodium intake is also important. By controlling these two factors you can control most of the toxins/waste created by your body and in turn, this helps your kidney function. If you catch this early enough and really moderate your diet with extreme care, you could prevent total renal failure. If you catch this early you can eliminate the problem completely.

RENAL DIET RECIPES

1. Lime Grilled Turkey Recipe

Prep Time: 15 mins Total Time: 40 mins

Servings: 4

Ingredients

- ½ cup (125 mL) lime juice
- 1 tsp (5 mL) rosemary, dried
- ¼ cup (60 mL) vegetable oil
- 2 tbsp (30 mL) honey, liquid

1 tsp (5 mL) thyme leaves, dried

⅔ lb (300 g) turkey breast, skinless, boneless

Directions:

1. Make the marinade by mixing the first five ingredients.
2. Set aside 2 tbsp (30 mL) of marinade for basting.
3. Slice turkey breast in half lengthwise to make thinner pieces (like a hamburger bun is cut in half).
4. Add turkey to marinade and place in the fridge for 1 – 2 hours.
5. Preheat oven broiler on high (500°F) or preheat barbeque.
6. Broil or grill the turkey for 4 minutes per side until cooked through.
7. Use marinade set aside in step 2 to baste the turkey while cooking.

8. Throw out the leftover marinade.

2. Kickin' Chicken Tacos Recipe

Prep Time: 10 mins Total Time: 25 mins

Servings: 4

 Ingredients

1 pound boneless, skinless chicken breasts

1 1/2 teaspoons salt-free taco seasoning

2 green onions (scallions), sliced

1 lime, juiced

8 corn tortillas

1 cup iceberg lettuce, shredded or chopped

1/4 cup sour cream

1/2 cup cilantro, chopped

Directions:

1. Boil chicken for 20 minutes.

2. Shred chicken into bite-size pieces or chop finely.

3. Toss chicken with Mexican seasoning and lime juice.

4. Fill tortillas with chicken and lettuce.

5. Top with sour cream, green onions, cilantro or other garnishes.

3. Shrimp and Apple Stir Fry Recipe

Prep Time: 15 mins Total Time: 35 mins

Servings: 4

Ingredients

1/2 lb (227 g) Headless shrimp with shells

3/4 Apple, diced

2 Celery stalks, diced

1/2 Sweet red pepper, diced

2 tbsp (30 mL) Vegetable oil

Marinade

1/2 tsp (2.5 mL) Low sodium soy sauce

1 tsp (5 mL) Cornstarch   Dash of White pepper

Sauce

1/2 tsp (2.5 mL) Low sodium soy sauce

1 tsp (5 mL) Sugar

1   tsp (5 mL) Cornstarch

2   tbsp (30 mL) Coldwater Directions:

1. Remove shells and devein shrimp. Marinade the shrimp using the

1.   marinade ingredients listed above for half an hour.

2.   Combine sauce ingredients in a small bowl. Mix well and set aside.

212

3.   Heat about 1 tablespoon of oil in a non-stick wok. Stir fry shrimp until the shrimp turns pink in color, remove from the wok.

4.   Heat about 1 tablespoon of oil in a non-stick wok. Stir fry celery briefly, and then add the diced apple and red pepper, stirring until almost cooked through. Add in the shrimp and the sauce mixture and stir constantly until the sauce thickens. Ready to serve.

4. Low Salt Stir-Fry Recipe

Prep Time: 10 mins Total Time: 20 mins

Servings: 2

Ingredients

- 4 cups (about 3/4 pound) mixed greens (lettuce, collard, beet, etc)

- 1 tablespoon olive oil

- 1 cup onions, sliced thin

- 1/4 teaspoon curry powder

- 1 tablespoon low sodium soy sauce

1/2 cup white wine vinegar or rice vinegar

8 ounces tofu, cut into cubes

1/2 teaspoon sesame oil

1/2
teaspoo
n
sesame
seeds

Directio
ns:

1. Cut greens into 2 inch long shreds.

2. Heat oil in a wok or saute pan.

3. Saute onions until translucent, about 2 minutes.

4. Sprinkle curry over onions and add sugar and greens.

5. Cover.

6. Reduce heat and let greens steam in their own juice until tender, 5-8 minutes. (During this time, uncover and turn occasionally. Add a little water if sticking.) Don't overcook or greens will turn darker.

7. Remove greens with a slotted spoon leaving juices in the pan.

8. Add soy sauce and vinegar, heat to boiling.

9. When the sauce is slightly thickened, remove from heat and pour over greens.

10. Garnish with sesame oil and seeds.

5. Orange-Glazed Chicken Recipe

Prep Time: 10 mins Total Time: 40 mins

Servings: 6

Ingredients

1/4 cup oil

6 chicken breast halves

2 tablespoons flour

1/8 teaspoon nutmeg

1 dash ginger

1/4 teaspoon cinnamon

1 1/2 cup orange Juice

1/4 cup raisins

1/2 cup mandarin orange (optional) Directions:

1.   Heat oil in a non-stick large fry pan.

2.   Brown chicken on both sides.

3.   Remove chicken and set aside.

4.   Blend flour, nutmeg, ginger, and cinnamon together; add the mixture to hot oil.

5.   Whisk together quickly to make a smooth paste.

6.   Gradually add orange juice to the pan.

7.   Stir constantly.

8.   Cook over medium heat until soft and thicken for 3 minutes.

9.   Return chicken to pan.

10.   Add raisins, cook on low heat for 30 minutes or until chicken is tender and fully cooked.

11.   If the sauce is too thick add water.

12.   Add mandarin orange slice and heat until warm.

6. Chicken Fusilli Salad Recipe

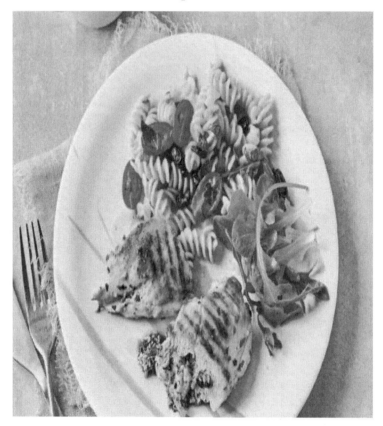

Prep Time: 10 mins Total Time: 30 mins

Servings: 4

Dressing

- 1/2 cup olive oil
-
-
-
-

220

1/4 cup vinegar

1/2 teaspoon white pepper

1/4 teaspoon basil

1 teaspoon sugar

Salad

3 cups cooked fusilli pasta (any pasta shape will work)

8 ounces cold cooked chicken, diced

1/2 cup frozen peas, defrosted

1/2cup chopped the red pepper

1 cup sliced zucchini

1 medium carrot, sliced thinly

2 cups shredded lettuce

Directions:

1. Put dressing ingredients in a jar with a lid and shake to blend ingredients. Chill for at least 2 hours. Shake again before mixing with salad.

2. Mix together pasta, chicken, peas, zucchini, red pepper and carrot in a large bowl.

3. Add dressing and toss well. Divide lettuce onto 4 plates and top with salad mixture.

7. Lemon Curry Chicken Salad Recipe

Prep Time: 15 mins Total Time: 25 mins

Servings: 4

Ingredients

1/4 cup vegetable oil

1/4 cup frozen lemonade concentrate, thawed

1/4 teaspoon ground ginger

1/4 teaspoon curry powder

1/8 teaspoon garlic powder

1 1/2 cups chicken, cooked and diced

1 1/2 cups grapes, halved

1/2 cup celery, sliced

Directions:

1.	In a large bowl, whisk together oil, lemonade concentrate, and spices.

2.	Add remaining ingredients and toss lightly.

3.	Chill at least an hour.

8. Braised beef with tomatoes and spring onions Recipe

Prep Time: 20 mins Total Time: 1 hr 15 mins

Servings: 4

Ingredients:

2tbsp groundnut oil

100g sliced celery

1 bay leaf

1tbsp tomato puree

8 tomatoes, roughly chopped

140ml red wine

500g large sliced stewing steak

200g chopped tinned tomatoes

1 onion, finely chopped

1 sprig rosemary   2 cloves garlic, crushed

200g shredded spring onions

1-liter beef stock

1tbsp chopped parsley

100g peeled diced carrots

Mashed potatoes, to serve

Directions:

1.   Heat the oil in a large pan. Add the beef in batches and fry to a good color. Take out and keep to one side.

2.   Add the onion and garlic to the oil to start to color. Add the tomato puree and stir, then add the wine and reduce by two-thirds.

3.   Put the beef back in and add the stock, carrots, celery and tinned tomatoes. Add the herb and bring to the boil.

4.   Simmer with the lid on for approximately 1¼ hours until just cooked.

5.   Carefully take out just the meat and keep warm. Pass the sauce through a liquidizer and then a strainer. Return to the pan and add the meat, finish cooking.

6.   Add the roughly chopped tomatoes and ¾ of the spring onions. Cook for a further minute.

7.   Serve sprinkled with parsley, the rest of the spring onions and mashed potatoes.

9. Zucchini Provencal Recipe

Prep Time: 10 mins Total Time: 25 mins

Servings: 6

Ingredients

2 potatoes

5 large zucchini

1   cup celery, chopped

2   red bell pepper

2 tomatoes

1/2 cup green onions, chopped

1/2 teaspoon basil

2 tablespoons oil

3   Directions:

1.   Dice potatoes into 1/2 inch pieces and cut zucchini into 1-inch chunks.

2.   Slice bell peppers.

3.   If using whole tomatoes, quarter and slice through again.

4.   In a large pan, saute onions, basil, and celery in oil.

5.   Add tomatoes, zucchini, and potatoes.

6.   Stir gently, then cover and steam until tender.

10. Easy Paella Recipe

Prep Time: 10 mins Total Time: 30 mins

Servings: 6 - 8

Ingredients

1 tablespoon olive oil

1 cup yellow onion, chopped

1 1/2 cups low sodium chicken broth

2 jars roasted red peppers, pureed

1/2 teaspoon paprika

1/2 teaspoon Tabasco sauce

1/2 pound Italian sausage

1/2 pound chicken breast, diced

1-2 garlic cloves, pressed

2 cups uncooked short grain rice

10 strands or 1/8 teaspoon saffron

1/2 pound shrimp, uncooked, shelled, deveined

1/2 cup each red and green peppers, sliced in strips

1/2 cup frozen green peas

Directions:

1. Heat olive oil in a large pan and saute sausage, chicken, and garlic until meat is browned.

2. Remove meats and set aside.

3. Add rice and onion to the pan and saute until onion is translucent and rice is golden brown.

4. Add meat back to pan with broth and pureed red bell peppers.

5. Add paprika, Tabasco, and saffron.

6. Bring to a boil; reduce heat to low, and simmer covered for 10 minutes.

7. Stir in shrimp, bell peppers, and peas.

8. Cover and cook 10 minutes.

11. Breakfast Burritos with Eggs and Mexican Sausage Recipe

Prep Time: 15 mins Total Time: 25 mins

Servings: 3

Ingredients

3 ounces of chorizo (Mexican sausage)

3 flour tortillas

3 eggs, beaten Directions:

1.   Fry chorizo in the skillet until dark in color.

2.   Add eggs and cook until done.

3.   Fill warmed tortillas with mixture and roll up, folding up the bottom edge before rolling to keep the filling from falling out.

12. Alaska Baked Macaroni and Cheese Recipe

Prep Time: 15 mins Total Time: 30 mins

Servings: 8

Ingredients

3 cups elbow, small shell or bowtie pasta

2 tablespoons flour

1 tablespoon fresh thyme or tarragon, chopped or 1 teaspoon dry

2 cups cheese (gouda, cheddar, or any combo)

2 tablespoons unsalted butter

2 cups of milk

1 teaspoon mustard powder   1 teaspoon paprika

croutons or chopped almonds to taste Directions:

1. Heat oven to 350 degrees.

2. Boil pasta in a large pot until al-dente.

3.   Meanwhile, in a medium glass measuring cup, measure flour and butter. Microwave about 1-2 minutes until golden brown.

4.   Slowly stir in milk and continue microwaving until thickened. Stir in spices and herbs.

5.   Mix drained noodles, sauce, and cheese and put in a greased casserole dish. Bake about 20 minutes.

6.   Top with croutons or chopped almonds in the last 5 minutes.

13.   Italian Eggplant Salad Recipe

14.

Prep Time: 10 mins Total Time: 30 mins

Servings: 4

Ingredients

3 cups cubed eggplant

1 small onion, chopped

1   medium tomato, chopped

2   tablespoons white wine vinegar

1 clove garlic, chopped

1/2 teaspoon oregano

1/4 teaspoon black pepper

3 tablespoons olive oil

Directions:

1. Add eggplant to boiling water in a saucepan.
2. Reheat to boiling; reduce heat.
3. Cover and cook until tender, about 10 minutes; drain.
4. Place eggplant and onion in a glass dish.
5. Mix together vinegar, garlic, and pepper.
6. Pour over eggplant and onion; toss.
7. Stir in oil just before serving.

14. Chilli Con Carne Recipe

Prep Time: 15 mins Total Time: 55 mins

Servings: 4

Ingredients:

- 200g/8oz canned red kidney beans in water, rinsed and drained

- 1 medium onion, chopped

- ½ teaspoon chili powder, or more to taste

200g/8ox tinned tomatoes

½ teaspoon paprika

½ tablespoon vinegar

1 clove garlic, crushed

1 tablespoon vegetable oil

500g/1lb minced beef, low fat, if possible

½ tablespoon sugar (optional)

Directions:

1. Heat the oil over low heat and fry onion and garlic for about five minutes

2. Add the minced beef and fry until lightly browned

3. Add all the other ingredients, except the kidney beans, and mix together. Simmer gently on the hob for about 30 minutes, adding a little extra water if necessary 4. Add the kidney beans and cook for a further 10 minutes

5. Serve with rice and crusty bread or green side salad.

15. Mini Pineapple Upside Down Cakes Recipe

Prep Time: 15 mins Total Time: 35 mins

Servings: 12

Ingredients

    3 tablespoons unsalted butter, melted

    1/3 cup packed brown sugar

    12 canned unsweetened pineapple slices

    1-1/3 cups cake flour

1-1/4 teaspoons baking powder

6 fresh cherries cut into halves and pitted

2/3 cup sugar

2/3 cup fat-free milk

3 tablespoons canola oil   1 egg

1 teaspoon lemon juice

1/2 teaspoon vanilla extract

1/4 teaspoon salt

Directions:

1. Sprinkle a little brown sugar into each section.

2. Press one pineapple slice into each section forming a cup shape. Place one cherry half (cut side facing up) in the center of each pineapple slice and set aside.

3. In a large bowl, beat the sugar, milk, oil, egg, and extracts until well blended. Combine the flour, baking powder, and salt; gradually beat into sugar mixture until blended. Pour into prepared batter into muffin pan.

4. Bake at 350° for 35-40 minutes or until a toothpick comes out clean. Immediately invert the muffin pan

and drop the cooked cakes onto a serving plate. You can use a butter knife or small spatula along the edges if necessary to gently release them from the pan. Serve warm.

16. Speedy Tortilla Wraps Recipe

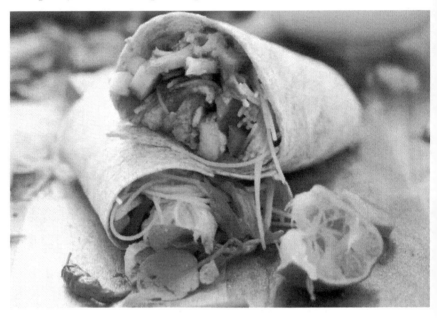

Prep Time: 15 mins Total Time: 40 mins

Servings: 6

+ Ingredients
+
+ 4 ounces cream cheese
+
+ 1 red bell pepper, sliced
+
3 7" flour or corn tortillas

1 cup lettuce

4 ounces leftover chicken, beef or fish

1 tablespoon mayonnaise or
low   sodium   ranch

Directions:

1. Spread cream cheese on tortilla.

2. Lay on lettuce leaves, meat, and pepper slices.

3. Spread with mayonnaise or low sodium ranch dressing.

4. Roll up each tortilla like a jelly roll.

5. Cut in half and wrap in plastic wrap to hold together.

6. Keep chilled in cooler for 6-8 hours.

17. Lemon and ginger baked yogurt chicken with fresh curry leaves Recipe

Prep Time: 35 mins Cooking Time: 20-25 mins Total Time: 55 mins - 1 hr

Servings: 4

Ingredients:

- 1 free range chicken portioned into 8 pieces (2 thighs, 2 drumsticks, 2 winglets, and 2 breasts)

- 1 lemon juice plus zest (approx 50ml)

- 150/100ml natural yogurt

- 10 twists of black peppercorns

- 15g garlic

- 15g ginger

- 1/2 tsp of cumin seed

- 1/4 tsp ground coriander

- 1/2 fresh red chili approx 5g

- 10 fresh curry leaves

Directions:

1. Make incisions into the flesh with a sharp knife as this will help to make it cook quicker and also allow the spice to permeate right into the meat.

2. Place all of the ingredients, except the yogurt, into a food processor and blend until fine.

3. Remove the spice mixture from blender and mix into the chicken thoroughly.

4. Then add the yogurt. Ideally, leave in the fridge for 24 hours.

5. Pre-heat oven to 220 degrees and place chicken pieces on a foil-lined tray.

6. Bake for approx 20/25 mins.

7. Remove from the oven and serve with some plain rice.

18. Thai Lettuce Wraps Recipe

Prep Time: 10 mins Total Time: 30 mins

Servings: 6

⊥ Ingredients
⊥
⊥   1   tablespoon vegetable oil
⊥
⊥   1/2 teaspoon shrimp paste
⊥
⊥   2   teaspoons granulated sugar
⊥
⊥   4 tablespoons fresh cilantro, finely chopped
⊥
⊥   249
⊥
⊥

3 green onions or shallots, thinly sliced

1 Thai chili, diced

3 garlic cloves, minced

1 1/2 pounds ground pork

1 tablespoon Homemade Low Sodium Soy Sauce

3 tablespoons fresh basil, finely chopped

8 leaves iceberg or butter lettuce

Directions:

1. Heat oil in a large skillet or wok over medium heat.

2. Add green onions, Thai chili, and garlic.

3. Stir-fry for 2 minutes.

4. Add ground pork and cook for 15 minutes or until cooked through.

5. Add low sodium soy sauce, shrimp paste, sugar, and a half each of the cilantro and basil.

6. Cook for 5 minutes.

7. Top with remaining cilantro and basil.

8. Fill lettuce leaves with about 2 ounces of pork mixture.

Antony Jason Willfour

19. BBQ Corn on the Cob Recipe

Prep Time: 10 mins Total Time: 35 mins

Servings: 8

- Ingredients
-
- 3 tablespoons olive oil
-
- 1/2 teaspoon black pepper
-
1 tbs grated parmesan cheese

1 tsp teaspoon dried thyme

1 tsp parsley

4 fresh corn on the cob, cut into 8 halves

Directions:

1. Husk and clean the corn (or you can buy 4 prepped ears from the produce section of the store).

2. Mix the oil, cheese, thyme, parsley and black pepper in a dish wide enough to roll the corn into and completely cover with mixture.

3. Place the corn in the mixture and roll to thoroughly coat corn.

4. Place all of the corn onto the center of a heavy-duty aluminum foil sheet.

5. Fold up the edges of the foil sheet to create a tray making sure not to leave space for the oil to drip onto the grill.

6. Place the foil tray on the grill over medium heat and cook for 15-20 minutes turning as browning is done one each side.

20. Wild Rice Stuffing Recipe

Prep Time: 15 mins Total Time: 30 mins

Servings: 8-10

Ingredients

2 cups uncooked wild rice

1/4 cup butter or margarine

1 cup water chestnuts, diced

1 cup shelled pistachio nuts

4 cups low sodium turkey, chicken or mushroom broth

2 cups mushrooms, sliced

1 onion, chopped

1 cup dried apricots, chopped

1 cup dried cherries, chopped

1/4 cup fresh or 1 teaspoon dried thyme

1/4 cup fresh or 1 teaspoon dried tarragon

Directions:

1. Cook 2 cups wild rice in low sodium turkey, chicken, or mushroom broth.
2. Preheat oven to 350 degrees.
3. Saute mushrooms, onion, apricots, cherries in butter.
4. Add water chestnuts, pistachios and rice. Cook, stirring, for about 5 minutes.
5. Add herbs and place in the greased baking dish and bake about 30 minutes.

6. A great side dish to turkey at Thanksgiving or with a roast chicken. You can double or triple the recipe and freeze it, it keeps well for months.

21. Pancakes with easy toffee sauce Recipe

Prep Time: 15 mins Total Time: 5 mins

Servings: 4

Ingredients:

100g plain flour

300ml milk

50g (2oz) granulated sugar   1 tbsp sunflower or vegetable oil,   plus a little extra for frying

150g (2oz) golden syrup

50g (2oz) butter

2 large eggs

75g (3oz) soft brown sugar

150ml (5 fl oz) double cream   A few drops vanilla extract
Directions:

1.   Put the flour, eggs, milk into a bowl and whisk to a smooth batter. Set aside for 30 mins to rest if you have time, or start cooking straight away.

2.   Set a medium frying pan over medium heat and carefully wipe it with some oiled kitchen paper. When hot, cook your pancakes for 1 min on each side until golden, keeping them warm in a low oven as you go.

3.   Toffee sauce method:

4.   Place the butter, sugars, and syrup in a saucepan and, over very low heat, allow everything to dissolve completely. Let it cook for about 5 minutes.

5.   Pour in the cream and vanilla extract an'
everything is smooth. Remove it from the heat anu
to cool completely before pouring it into a jug ready for
serving.

6.   Serve on pancakes with ice cream..

22. Cornbread Muffins Recipe

Prep Time: 10 Total Time: 35 mins

Servings: 12

Ingredients

1 cup all-purpose flour

1/4 cup honey

1/2 cup buttermilk

1 cup cornmeal

1/2 teaspoon baking soda

1/4 cup granulated sugar

1/2 cup unsalted butter, softened   2 eggs

1/2 cup no salt added canned corn Directions:

1.   Preheat oven to 400 degrees.

2.   Use a cooking oil spray to lightly grease a muffin pan.

3.   In a large bowl, combine flour, cornmeal, baking soda, and sugar.

4.   Mix in butter using a pastry blender or mix in a food processor until butter is pea-sized.

5.   In a separate bowl, beat eggs.

6.   Mix in honey and buttermilk.

7.   Pour egg mixture into the flour mixture stirring until just mixed.

8.   Fold in the corn.

9.   Spoon batter into muffin cups and bake for 20-25 minutes or until a toothpick inserted into the center of a muffin comes out clean.

23. Mediterranean Pizza Recipe

Prep Time: 15 mins Total Time: 30 mins

Servings: 12

Ingredients

1 crust, 2 pitas ready-made pizza dough or large pitas

1 Roma tomato, sliced

10 basil leaves, thinly sliced

1   tablespoon olive oil

2   garlic cloves, sliced thinly

3   ounces goat cheese, or ricotta Directions:

1.   Preheat oven to 450 degrees.

2.   Coat pizza crust with olive oil.

3.   Arrange garlic slices evenly across the crust.

4.   Cover garlic with tomato slices.

5.   Sprinkle basil evenly over pizza then top with goat cheese.

6.   Bake in the oven for 10-15 minutes or as otherwise directed by crust package instructions.

24. Chicken and Orange Salad Sandwich Recipe

Prep Time: 10 mins Total Time: 20 mins

Servings: 6

Ingredients

1 cup chopped cooked chicken

1/2 cup green pepper, chopped

1/4 cup onion, finely sliced

1 cup Mandarin oranges

1/2 cup celery, diced

1/3 cup mayonnaise Directions:

1.   Toss chicken, celery, green pepper, and onion to mix.

2.   Add mandarin oranges and mayonnaise.

3.   Mix gently.

4.   Serve on bread. Enjoy.

25. Chicken Seafood Gumbo Recipe

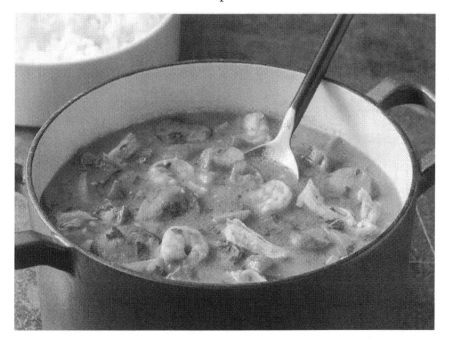

Prep Time: 15 mins Total Time: 35 mins

Servings: 12

Ingredients

1 tablespoon canola oil

3 celery stalks, chopped

1 yellow onion, chopped

1   red bell pepper, chopped

2   skinless chicken breasts, chopped

8 ounces lean smoked turkey sausage, sliced

1/2 cup canola oil

1/2 cup flour

1   tablespoon salt-free Cajun seasoning

2   quarts low sodium chicken broth

1/2 pound cooked shrimp

6 ounces canned crab, drained

3 cups frozen okra, chopped Directions:

1.   Heat 1 tablespoon canola oil in a 4.5 quart or larger pot over medium heat.

2.   Add celery, onion, bell pepper, chicken, and sausage and cook for 10 minutes.

3.   Remove mixture from pot and set aside.

4.   Reduce heat to medium.

5.   Add 1/2 cup canola oil and stir in flour to make a roux.

6.   Stir in Cajun seasoning and let cook for a minute or more depending on how dark you want your gumbo to be.

7.   Very slowly stir in chicken broth, stirring constantly to avoid lumps.

8.   Increase heat to medium-high and bring mixture to a boil and let boil for about 10 minutes or until it starts to thicken slightly.

9.   Reduce heat to medium and add shrimp, crab, and okra, and add the chicken mixture back into the pot as well.

10.   Cook for 10 minutes or until heated through.

CONCLUSION

Renal diets are designed to help those suffering from kidney disease to live a better, more healthy life.

Certain types of food can be detrimental to abnormal kidneys, so make sure to have a good working knowledge of not only the disease but also how it affects your body specifically. Many people look at kidney disease as the end of life. In truth, this sort of diet helps you manage your health and keep your kidney disease at bay.

Your doctor can give you many more pointers than this article, and should always be consulted or notified of any change in your condition. If you have renal issues these diets are essential to managing your health and helping you to feel better.

Dietitians have experience working with those suffering from renal issues and can give some general guidelines to follow, such as:

+ Limit Intake of Potassium- Apples, strawberries, broccoli, cabbage, cauliflower are on the list of things that are low in Potassium.

✦ Limit Intake of Phosphorous- Pasta, rice, corn-based cereals, and liquid non-dairy creamer are on the OK list.

✦ Limit Fluid Intake- 48 ounces of fluid per day is the recommended limit for renal diets- be sure to count the fluid in things like grapes, ice cream, oranges, etc.

✦ Limit Intake of Salt- You'll need to be a label reader to make sure you keep your sodium intake down- know what you are putting into your body and the effect it may have.

✦ Limit Intake of Protein- Between 5 and 7 ounces of protein per day is the limit for a renal diet. Using egg substitutes instead of regular eggs is a good way to keep your protein intake low.

If you decide to work with a dietitian, they can point you precisely to what you should and should not eat and why. Knowing the effect food has on your body is powerful knowledge and can help how you feel on a day to day basis. Certainly, every case is different and you should always talk to your doctor. But renal diets have helped many sufferers of kidney disease to get and stay healthier.

Made in the USA
Middletown, DE
12 October 2020